Po ~

John P. Vance, M.D., F.F.A.R.C.S., D. Obst. R.C.O.G.
and
Agnes Corrigan, M.A., M.Sc., R.G.N.

William Heinemann Medical Books Ltd
London

First published by William Heinemann Medical Books Ltd
23 Bedford Square, London WC1B 3HH 1983

ISBN 0-433-33647-1

Printed in Great Britain by Henry Ling Ltd., at the Dorset Press,
Dorchester, Dorset

Contents

Acknowledgements

The help of the Medical Illustration Departments at Canniesburn Hospital Plastic Surgery Unit and at the Royal Infirmary, Glasgow, is gratefully acknowledged. We are also grateful to Mr D. S. Soutar for his ready agreement to our publishing photographs of certain of his patients and to those patients themselves for their cooperation. Sister G. Shanley, Sister in Charge of the Recovery Room at the Plastic Surgery Unit, Canniesburn Hospital, modelled for many of the illustrations and we are indebted to her.

Finally, but very importantly, Miss Sheena Sandeman readily gave of her time and secretarial expertise in preparing the manuscript and we are most grateful to her.

Introduction

The concept of progressive patient care is now well established. Inherent in this concept is the idea that the more acutely or severely ill a patient is, the more staff and facilities should be provided for his care, and that equipment and appropriately experienced nursing and medical staff should be concentrated in specialised areas to provide this care. Thus, in recent years, we have seen an increase in numbers of such special areas as Intensive Care Units, Coronary Care Units, Renal Dialysis Units and Postoperative Recovery Areas.

When a patient undergoes surgery, it is probable that at no other time in his life will he have such a concentration of medical and nursing personnel directed towards his care, including the surgeon and his assistant dealing with the lesion to be operated on, the anaesthetist providing anaesthesia and looking after the patient's general well-being with special regard to his circulation and respiration, and the nursing staff providing instruments at the operating table as well as being responsible for the smooth running of the operating theatre.

Such a concentration of effort would be pointless if close attention were not continued into the postoperative period, and it is in this area of surgical care that some of the greatest advances have been made in the last 20 years. It is no longer acceptable for a patient to be wheeled back to his ward bed in an unconscious state and looked at only occasionally by the busy ward staff to ascertain that he is still breathing.

Nowadays it is vital that every patient who has had surgery should pass through a recovery area. Ideally this should be a special area or ward adjacent to the theatre suite. It should be suitably equipped and well staffed with nurses experienced in looking after patients in the immediate postoperative period. Although all recently-built hospitals have a specialised recovery area, it is unfortunate that many older hospitals do not. Many of these were built with their operating theatres on different floors and widely scattered throughout the hospital; it is therefore impossible for them to have a single recovery area because of problems of transporting patients to and from such an area and probably also because of shortage of suitable space. Nevertheless, a space should be provided where the patient may recover under close supervision. This may only be a room off the theatre corridor, but it should contain all the necessary equipment and be suitably staffed.

Although this book is based on the treatment of patients in a purpose-built recovery area, the principles stated apply to all patients in whatever kind of recovery facility is available.

Much of what is stated in this book is applicable throughout the whole of the patient's postoperative period; the main emphasis, however, has been placed on the immediate few hours following surgery. All patients deserve the very highest standard of care at all times but especially so at this very critical time in their hospital stay.

CHAPTER 1

The Recovery Room

Patients who have had all kinds of surgery, from the most minor to the most major, will be admitted to the recovery area after their operations. It follows therefore that staff, facilities and equipment for the care of such patients must be available.

The most important requirement is, undoubtedly, the presence of adequate numbers of well-trained nursing and medical staff to observe patients and treat them as necessary. Ideally it would be desirable to have a nurse for each recovery room bed. For most hospitals this would be an intolerable drain on numbers of nurses; a compromise would be one nurse for each patient who has had major, complex surgery, and one nurse between two patients having minor surgery.

A member of the medical staff should be constantly available to deal with medical problems arising within the area. This is often a member of the anaesthetic staff, but may be one of the surgical staff.

The number of beds in a recovery area will depend on the number of operating theatres served and on the throughput of patients from these theatres. For example, a cardiothoracic theatre may yield only two or three patients per day whereas a gynaecology theatre may provide a dozen or more minor cases who will, for the most part, be short-stay patients as far as the recovery area is concerned. As a rule, the more minor the surgery, the shorter the anaesthetic and the more rapidly the patient recovers consciousness and respiratory and cardiovascular stability. It should be noted from the previous statement that not only is recovery of consciousness postoperatively important but also the condition of the patient with regard to adequacy of breathing and stability of circulation. With modern techniques of anaesthesia, many patients will have regained consciousness by the time they reach the recovery room. If the patient is reasonably fit and the surgery has been minor, such a patient may only need to remain in the recovery area for a few minutes to allow checking of pulse, blood pressure and respiration before returning to the ward. On the other hand, although a patient who has had major surgery may rapidly regain consciousness, he may have suffered major blood loss and require fluid or further blood replacement to produce cardiovascular stability, or he may be hypothermic and need to be warmed. It may take a number of hours to attain the desired level of stability and, during this time, constant monitoring of many variables will be required. Not until these have reached satisfactory levels should the patient return to the ward.

Siting of Recovery Room

The recovery area must be adjacent to the theatre or theatres being served so that the distance and time taken in transporting patients from theatre to recovery area is as short as possible. This is important because, while a patient is being moved on a trolley, it is much less easy to observe his colour, breathing, pulse and other factors which indicate his state of well-being.

In the modern theatre suite, the theatres are usually contained within a 'clean area'; that is to say an area which is only entered by persons who are suitably dressed in theatre clothing and footwear. The recovery area should also be contained within this clean area; nursing and medical staff may then pass freely from theatres to recovery area without having to change clothing and the patient will not have to be transferred from a 'clean area' trolley to another trolley when he is moved to the recovery area. If the design of the theatre area is such that the recovery area is outside the 'clean area', the patient should be transferred from theatre trolley to his own bed for his stay in the recovery area.

Facilities in the Recovery Room

The recovery room will be divided into an appropriate number of 'bays', each of which will be equipped to receive a patient on his trolley or bed. The bays should be separated by curtains which can be drawn to provide privacy for nursing and medical procedures and withdrawn to allow easy observation of the patient. Each bay should be spacious enough to give easy access of staff to the patient and also room for bulky equipment such as a resuscitation trolley or mobile x-ray machine.

There should be an oxygen outlet and at least one, preferably two, vacuum points in each bay. Two vacuum sources are preferable since a patient may require suction to be applied continuously to a surgical drain while suction may also be required at the same time to remove secretions from the airway.

The oxygen and vacuum outlets will be in the wall at the head end of the bay and the apparatus for delivery of oxygen (*see* Chapter 6) or control of suction will usually be supported on the wall adjacent to the outlet. Often the support is provided by a bar, screwed to the wall, along which the various pieces of equipment can be moved until their position is suitable in relation to the patient.

The other very important facility which each bay requires is an adequate number of electrical outlets. At least six per bay should be available, since certain patients will require a number of items of electrical apparatus to be in use simultaneously. For example, a patient may require a pulmonary ventilator, an electrocardiograph monitor, a blood warmer, a drip controller or infusion pump and an electric blanket. Thus, it is easy to see why a large number of electrical outlets are required. Certain of these items of equipment, such as the ECG monitor, may also be supported on the bar mentioned above or, alternatively, small shelves or trolleys may be provided.

Many patients coming from theatre will have intravenous infusions running and some means of supporting drip bottles and bags must be available. This may be provided in the form of conventional drip stands but can be more conveniently provided by having poles suspended from rails on the ceiling along which the poles may slide. A rail should be provided along each side of the bay. Minimising the need for drip stands at the bedside allows easier access to the patient.

Equipment in the Recovery Room

From comments already made, it will be obvious that a large range of equipment will be needed in the recovery room. Much of this is described in the following chapters, but the variety of equipment required is listed below.

Equipment for airway management

Oropharyngeal and nasopharyngeal airways; tracheal tubes (oral and nasal); laryngoscopes; suction catheters and tubing.

Equipment for respiratory support

Ambu bag or similar type of manual device for artificial ventilation; automatic ventilators.

Equipment for oxygen therapy

Oxygen flow meters; humidifiers for oxygen; masks and tubing for delivery of oxygen to patient; 'T' pieces for connection of oxygen tubing to tracheal tubes.

Equipment for monitoring

Electrocardiograph; blood pressure (manual or direct); central venous pressure; temperature; urinary output.

Equipment for intravenous infusions

Supply of intravenous fluids; plasma substitutes; refrigerator for storing blood for transfusion; intravenous giving sets; intravenous cannulae; central venous catheters; drip controllers or infusion pumps; blood warmers; pressure infusors (for pressurising bags of intravenous fluid for rapid transfusion); blood filters.

General

Syringes and needles; swabs; preparations for cleaning skin prior to injections etc.; forms and appropriate sample tubes for biochemistry, haematology, blood transfusion, bacteriology; requirements for general nursing care, e.g. wound dressing materials, bed linen, pillows, bed pans, sick bowls, etc.

Resuscitation equipment

The requirements for resuscitation will have been covered in the foregoing list with the exception of drugs and a defibrillator but a separate trolley (Fig. 1.1) should be provided within the recovery area on which the following should be kept for emergency use.

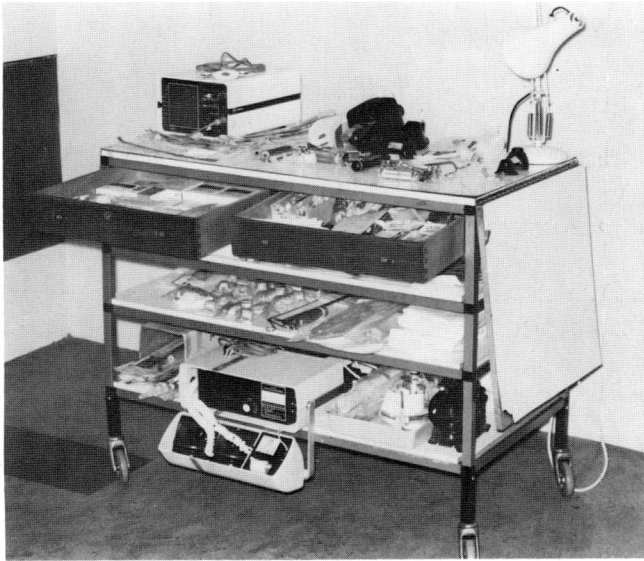

Fig. 1.1 *A resuscitation trolley. This carries all the equipment likely to be required for a patient needing emergency respiratory or cardiovascular support. Note the defibrillator on the bottom shelf. The lamp on the upper surface is fixed and stable. The flap on the right-hand side hinges upward to provide a working surface if required. Drugs are contained in the left-hand drawer and intravenous cannulae, needles, etc., in the right-hand drawer.*

Equipment for airway management

Oral and nasal airways, oral and nasal tracheal tubes; tracheal tube introducer; two laryngoscopes with a full range of blade sizes (infant to large adult); Ambu or similar type of bag for manual artificial ventilation of the lungs with suitable face masks. If small infants and children are dealt with a suitable range of sizes of equipment will be required (Fig. 1.2).

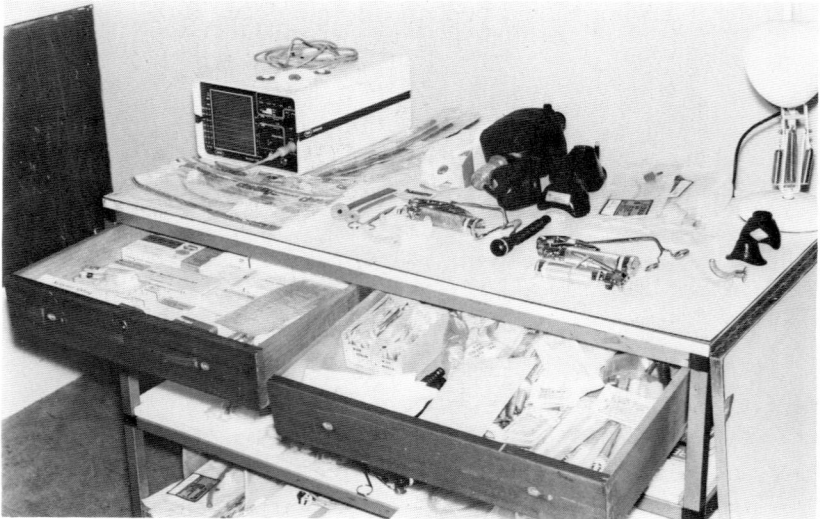

Fig. 1.2 *A closer view of the upper surface of the trolley in Fig. 1.1 shows the paediatric equipment on the right-hand side and the adult equipment on the left-hand side.*

Other equipment for resuscitation trolley

A *defibrillator* will be required; this must be kept fully charged by being plugged into an electrical supply when not in use (Fig. 1.3). Also required will be suction catheters, syringes and needles.

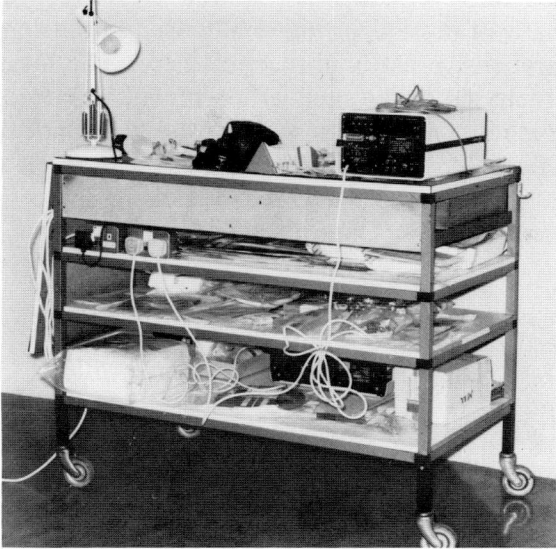

Fig. 1.3 *The back of the resuscitation trolley shows that it has an electrical power supply laid on. This is useful for providing power for the ECG monitor and the lamp and for keeping the defibrillator fully charged.*

Drugs for the resuscitation trolley

There will be a small range of drugs required in acute cardiac or respiratory emergencies: sodium bicarbonate solution 8.4%; adrenaline 1:1000; calcium chloride 10%; isoprenaline; atropine; lignocaine for intravenous use; a β-blocking drug, e.g. propranolol; a cardiac glycoside, e.g. Ouabain or digoxin; an antihistamine, e.g. promethazine; a bronchodilator, e.g. aminophylline; an anti-narcotic agent, e.g. naloxone; and also hydrocortisone. Sterile water for injection will also be required for dilution of drugs when necessary.

Drugs in the Recovery Room

In addition to the list of drugs required for acute resuscitation (a full supply of which should be available in addition to the emergency supply), a wide range of drugs is required in the recovery area and will include many of those drugs normally used in the surgical wards. Thus, a comprehensive list is impractical here. The most frequently used will be analgesic drugs such as morphine, papaveretum, pethidine, etc. A range of antibiotics will also be frequently used. Many other drugs will be required less frequently, for example local anaesthetic agents, insulin for diabetic patients, heparin, corticosteroids, diuretics and anti-emetics. Dantrolene should always be available (*see* Chapter 3).

The Recovery Room Bed or Trolley

The recovery room bed or trolley on which the patient is moved to the recovery room has certain fundamental requirements.

Firstly, it must be comfortable. This means having a mattress which is firm enough to support the patient, but soft enough to prevent discomfort from pressure on the hard metal trolley top. The mattress should also be washable. Usually such a mattress consists of a foam material covered by an impervious, non-slip, rubbery outer layer. It is usually about 75 cm in width, which is narrow enough to allow the trolley to be manoeuvrable but still gives sufficient width for comfort and allows the patient to be turned on his side. The need to turn the patient on his side means that the trolley must have sides which can be raised and lowered easily but, when raised, they must be sufficiently rigid to support the weight of the patient should he roll against them. The trolley must have a clearly recognisable head end and a mechanism which will allow it to be tilted rapidly into a head-down position. The non-slip quality of the mattress will prevent the patient from sliding towards the head end of the trolley when it is tilted. The trolley must also have a facility for carrying an oxygen cylinder and a shelf which can carry items such as a small portable suction apparatus, an 'Ambu' type resuscitator, airways, face masks and suction catheters.

The trolley must, of course, be mobile and the wheels of a suitable size. The wheels should be capable of being locked so as to stabilize the trolley for transferring the patient to and from the trolley and, since the trolley will have to be steered, the wheels should be capable of swivelling. Finally, the wheels should have solid rubber tyres, the rubber of which must be *anti-static*. This allows static electricity, which may build up in the trolley, to leak away through the floor and thus minimise the risk of sparking due to discharge of static electricity.

CHAPTER 2

General Nursing Management of the Postoperative Patient

The nursing care of the postoperative patient can be divided into two stages:

1. Immediate care either in the recovery room or ward.
2. Continuing care.

Immediate Care

Many hospitals now have a recovery room where the patient is under constant supervision by trained nursing staff. Patients who require continued specialised care are transferred to the intensive care unit. These are usually patients who

- are suffering from respiratory insufficiency;
- have undergone very major surgery;
- have had pre-operative respiratory and/or cardiac problems;
- have had intra-operative cardiorespiratory problems.

Whether the patient is in the recovery room or in a surgical ward, the principles of immediate care are the same. It is the responsibility of the nurse to ensure that all the equipment for postoperative care is available and ready for use before the patient returns from theatre. This includes an accessible oxygen supply with various types of oxygen masks, a functioning suction machine with a selection of sterile catheters, an airway, a sphygmomanometer and cuff, a stethoscope, a thermometer, and paper wipes and bowl. Labelled charts should also be available for charting the patient's blood pressure, pulse, respiratory rate, temperature and fluid balance. On receiving the patient from theatre, the nurse must find out from the anaesthetist and/or theatre nurse what type of operation was performed, whether there were any complications either due to the anaesthetic or to the surgical procedure, and whether the patient's condition is stable.

In the immediate care of the patient the following aims, which are discussed and developed further in the section on continuing care, must be realised.

AIM 1: To promote normal respiratory function

The nurse should observe the colour and warmth of the patient's skin. The level of consciousness of the patient must also be noted, for example, by using the patient's response to his name.

The patient's respiratory rate and depth of respirations should be recorded immediately and at intervals thereafter. Controlled oxygen therapy, if prescribed, is given (*see* Chapter 4).

AIM 2: To promote normal cardiovascular function

This is attained by monitoring the patient's blood pressure and pulse rate. These observations should be recorded immediately and every 15 minutes until the vital signs are stable. The nurse must ensure that the patient is moved carefully from the trolley to the bed, as rapid changes in position may predispose to hypotension.

AIM 3: To promote fluid and electrolyte balance

Intravenous infusions are observed for type of fluid and rate of flow. The intravenous site should be observed for inflammation and infiltration into the tissues. If a blood transfusion is in progress, the nurse should be aware of the signs of a possible reaction. The wound site is observed for colour, type and amount of drainage.

AIM 4: To promote normal renal function

If a bladder catheter is *in situ* the nurse must ensure it is unclamped and attached to a drainage bag.

Continuing Care

In this section the continuing care of the postoperative patient is discussed, using the four aims referred to above.

AIM 1: To promote normal respiratory function

To realise this aim, the nurse must ensure the maintenance of an open airway at all times following surgery.

In observing the patient the nurse should be aware that restlessness, confusion, rapid shallow breathing, gasping for air, cyanosis, respiratory stridor and wheezing are signs of obstruction. She should inform the doctor immediately if any of these signs are present.

The nurse can aid the promotion of normal respiratory function by:

a. Positioning the patient on his side until his swallowing and gag reflexes return.
b. Gently applying suction to the patient's mouth and throat to remove mucus and blood.
c. Leaving the oral airway in place until the patient pushes it out of his mouth himself.
d. If oxygen has been ordered, administering the prescribed amount and ensuring the patient receives this.
e. Sitting the patient up in bed as soon as his condition is stable and encouraging good lung ventilation by deep breathing. (After certain operations the surgeon may not wish the patient to sit up—this should be ascertained from the surgeon.)
f. Encouraging the patient to cough and observing the colour and consistency of the mucus he expectorates.

AIM 2: To promote normal cardiovascular function

To realise this aim, the nurse monitors the patient's blood pressure, pulse and respiratory rate.

Blood pressure

Normal blood pressure should be evaluated on an individual basis. The baseline is the patient's blood pressure reading before surgery. The nurse should inform the doctor in the following circumstances: if the patient's systolic blood pressure is below 90 mmHg; if the patient's systolic blood pressure falls by more than 20 mmHg; if the blood pressure is continually falling by 5–10 mmHg over several readings. *Hypotension* postoperatively can be due to the premedication, anaesthetic drugs, or poor lung ventilation; it can also be an indication of low cardiac output possibly due to haemorrhage.

Pulse

Normally a patient's pulse is slightly rapid immediately after operation. The nurse should report if the patient has a bradycardia—i.e. a pulse rate below 60 beats/min. If there are no other symptoms, the pulse rate will usually return to normal. A *tachycardia*—i.e. a rate of over 110 beats/min—should also be reported. This can be associated with haemorrhage, pyrexia, lack of oxygen or cardiac arrhythmias; it may also be due to patient anxiety and pain. Any irregularities in the pulse rate should be reported as these may be an indication of abnormal cardiac rhythms.

Respirations

The patient's *respiratory rate* is recorded and the pattern is observed. Recordings are made initially according to the anaesthetist's or surgeon's instructions and thereafter according to the individual patient's requirements. The frequency of recordings is decreased as the patient's condition improves and stabilises.

AIM 3: To promote fluid and electrolyte balance

Imbalances of fluid and electrolytes lead to problems of over- and under-hydration. The objectives of fluid therapy are therefore:

a. To give sufficient fluids to maintain blood volume. This ensures that the patient has an adequate blood pressure, adequate cardiac output and an adequate urinary flow. Dehydration postoperatively can be caused either by fluid deficiencies existing prior to surgery or excess postoperative losses due to sweating, wound or gastrointestinal drainage.
b. To prevent *fluid overload*, which can lead to pulmonary oedema and cardiac failure.

The causes of fluid overload are excessive administration of fluids or inadequate renal function. The nurse's responsibilities in helping to prevent fluid imbalance are:

● To record intake and output accurately.
● To administer the intravenous infusion or blood transfusion at the correct rate and on time.
● To record accurately the patient's central venous pressure if a central line is *in situ*.
● To report if the patient is suffering from severe prolonged vomiting.
● To observe and accurately chart drainage from gastric tubes, chest drains and wounds, and to ensure that drains do not become obstructed.

AIM 4: To promote normal renal function

Normally a patient should void urine within 8–10 hours following surgery. If the patient is adequately hydrated, inability to void may be due to pain, fear, tension or, in the case of the catheterised patient, the catheter not being patent.
A palpable fullness above the symphysis pubis or the frequent voiding of small amounts of urine are indications of bladder distension.

The nurse should attempt to relieve this by ensuring that the patient is pain free, in a comfortable position, and use stimuli such as running water and gentle manual pressure over the bladder area. Catheterisation should only rarely be required.

Accurate records of intake and output should be kept on all postoperative patients for at least the first 24 hours.

In some patients, especially those who have undergone urological surgery, urine volumes are measured hourly. If the volume falls below 30 ml in one hour, the doctor should be informed.

In considering the continuing care of the postoperative patient the promotion of homeostasis must realise the following aims:

AIM 5: To promote nutrition and elimination

The patient will receive intravenous fluids at first, then oral or nasogastric fluids and diet. If the patient is unable to take oral fluids, for example after major abdominal surgery, he may receive parenteral nutrition. Liquids will normally be given when the patient is no longer feeling nausea and he will then progress to a semi-solid diet. A full diet will be given as soon as the patient is able to tolerate it.

The patient should have a bowel movement by the second or third postoperative day and, if not, an aperient, suppositories or enema will be given.

AIM 6: To promote rest and comfort

Rest and sleep are essential for the patient's return to normal. To rest adequately, the patient must be free from pain. The intensity of postoperative pain is related to the patient's level of anxiety, his preoperative preparation and the extent of the surgical procedure.

Pain-relieving drugs are prescribed by a doctor; during the first 24 hours after the operation they are often given every 4–6 hours by intramuscular injection. Pain-relieving drugs may also be given by continuous intravenous infusion or via an epidural catheter.

The nurse should be aware of the possible complications of over-medication, such as respiratory depression.

Before administering the drugs, the nurse should:

a. Carefully read the prescription with another trained nurse.
b. Record the patient's blood pressure and, if it is low, inform the doctor (especially if the drug is being given by epidural catheter).
c. Observe the patient's conscious level and respiratory rate.
d. Look for the presence of any other problems, e.g. pressure points if the patient has a splint, abdominal distension, flatulence and hiccoughs.

After 24–48 hours postoperatively, a less potent drug is usually prescribed and given by the oral route if the patient is allowed oral intake.

If the patient continues to ask for pain-relieving drugs at frequent intervals several days after the operation the nurse should inform the doctor as this may be a sign of a *postoperative complication* developing. The nurse must observe for factors other than pain which cause the patient to be restless and agitated. These include bladder and abdominal distension, fear and *anxiety*, lack of oxygen, wet tight dressings and haemorrhage. The patient will also be uncomfortable if *nausea* and *vomiting* persist, which may be relieved by anti-emetics and sedatives. The nurse can help to prevent this situation by adequate preparation of the patient both mentally and physically during the pre-operative period. The nurse can promote freedom from anxiety in the patient by making him as comfortable as possible, by giving careful explanations at all times, and by listening to the patient's fears and anxieties. The patient will also be less anxious if he knows that his family have been informed of his condition.

As soon as possible, the patient should be placed in a comfortable position, have his face and hands washed, his hair brushed, and be given a clean gown and linen. *Mouth care* is important in all postoperative patients as they have often been given drugs to dry up their oral secretions. When the patient has recovered consciousness a mouth-wash is given and his teeth are cleaned. Special attention to mouth care is essential to prevent infection in patients who have undergone oral surgery.

AIM 7: To promote wound healing

Asepsis during surgery and in the postoperative period is the most important single factor in the promotion of wound healing. To achieve healing and prevent infection, which disrupts the process of wound repair, the wound may be covered with a sterile dressing, depending on the policy of the surgeon. If the wound is draining heavily, or where it is in a position to become contaminated by urine or faeces, then the dressings will require changing more often. The nurse should follow aseptic techniques when applying dressings.

Drains may be present in the wound:

a. When the area operated on has been contaminated with harmful collections of fluid, e.g. bile, pus, bowel contents, urine, pancreatic juice, all of which cause tissue irritation.
b. When there is a heavy blood loss and it must be measured accurately. When a large amount of fluid is present the drainage tube is often attached to low pressure suction. The nurse must ensure that the tubing is not twisted or kinked.
c. When a fistula-forming tube is required, for example, a 'T' tube or gastrostomy tube. These must be handled with care. If they are accidentally removed, irritant infective fluids will leak into the peritoneal cavity.

The nurse's responsibility in wound care also includes observing the wound for any signs of inflammation and reporting any elevation in the patient's temperature as these may indicate signs of infection.

AIM 8: To promote early ambulation and to return the patient to normality as soon as possible

The nurse should give passive exercises to the patient's limbs at frequent intervals until the patient is awake and, if the patient is critically ill, these should be continued.

Active exercises should begin as soon as the patient is awake.

The *physiotherapist* will have instructed the patient in the pre-operative period and the nurse should encourage him to move, turn, and flex arms and legs repeatedly while he is still confined to bed. *Deep breathing exercises* are also encouraged.

As soon as the surgeon permits, the patient is allowed to sit at the bedside and later, to be mobile. This is usually within a day or two of operation. The nurse must take special care of drains and infusions when the patient is getting up to sit or walk.

The patient should be encouraged to assume his own personal care as soon as possible.

Convalescence and Discharge

The patient's length of stay in hospital depends on:

1. His physical and mental health before surgery.
2. The extent of the operation.
3. Whether *postoperative complications* develop.
4. Arrangements at home for convalescence.
5. Community services available.

Before discharge, the nurse and the patient should have a knowledge of all of those factors.

In a patient whose operation has resulted in permanently changed body functions, for example if the patient has a permanent *colostomy*, the nurse must ensure that he is as independent as possible by teaching him how to care for and manage his changed physical function. There are many organisations and services which can help and advise the patient as well as giving continuing support. It is the nurse's responsibility to contact the relevant services before the patient is discharged.

AIM 9: To observe and prevent postoperative complications

Postoperative complications include:

haemorrhage
septicaemia
chest infections
wound infections and dehiscence
urinary infections
deep venous thrombosis
paralytic ileus

If the nurse has realised the previous aims, she will have prevented or have observed these complications in their early stages.

CHAPTER 3

Postoperative Observation and Monitoring

The length of stay in the recovery room and the amount of *monitoring* required will largely depend on the nature and duration of the surgery carried out and on the patient's previous health. For example, the healthy young woman who has had a minor gynaecological procedure, such as dilatation and curettage carried out without surgical or anaesthetic complications, will require at most, one or two checks on pulse, blood pressure and respirations and, assuming she has recovered consciousness, she will be ready for return to her ward about 15–30 minutes after entering the recovery area. This straightforward case can be contrasted with the elderly patient suffering from hypertension and chronic heart disease who has undergone emergency aortic graft surgery for a ruptured abdominal aortic aneurysm. Such a patient will be seriously ill, will have suffered major blood loss and transfusion of large volumes of blood and other fluids, and has a cardiac problem as well. The patient is also likely to be suffering from a certain degree of *hypothermia* postoperatively because a long operation, with a large abdominal incision and exposure of much of the abdominal contents, will result in the body temperature falling. Because of the large blood transfusion, a blood coagulation defect may occur, and if the illness has been associated with a period of low blood pressure, as it is almost certain to be, there may be a danger of renal failure. This patient obviously requires intensive monitoring of many functions including cardiovascular, respiratory, renal, haematological and biochemical, as well as observation of the lower limb circulation to ascertain adequate function of the aortic graft and observation of abdominal girth to help give an indication of intra-abdominal bleeding. Such a seriously ill patient may need to remain in the recovery room for many hours and may indeed require subsequent transfer to the intensive care unit for further management.

The variety of functions which can be monitored or observed are considered under several headings. Observations should be made and charted at regular intervals; the less stable the patient's condition the more frequent should be the observations. Accurate charting shows changes over a period and it is the trends thus demonstrated which may be of importance. Any observations made must be interpreted with regard to the patient's normal pre-operative findings.

Cardiovascular System

Pulse rate

The pulse rate is one of the fundamental cardiovascular observations. The normal rate depends on the age of the patient; it is between 120–140 beats per minute for infants and very young children, and 55–90 for the healthy resting adult. It may be influenced by drugs and may be excessively slow in certain heart conditions, for example, heart block.

An increasing heart rate during the postoperative period must always indicate the possibility of *haemorrhage*, especially when the operation has been inside one of the body cavities (abdomen or chest) and the bleeding cannot be seen. A rising pulse rate may also indicate inadequate pain relief and occasionally, *hypoxia*.

Blood pressure

Blood pressure should be measured and recorded at the same time as pulse rate. In a previously normotensive adult patient, a systolic pressure of not less than 90 mmHg would be regarded as acceptable. A figure of not less than 80 mmHg would be acceptable for a young child. The blood pressure may be low due to the effects of drugs administered during anaesthesia and normally this form of hypotension will respond to a rapid infusion of an appropriate intravenous fluid such as Hartmann's solution, *normal saline*, or *plasma*.

A falling blood pressure must always raise the suspicion of haemorrhage especially if associated with a rising pulse rate.

The blood pressure may be high as a result of inadequately treated pain. This is often associated with restlessness and a rapid pulse rate.

Blood pressure is most often measured indirectly by the method of Riva Rocci using a sphygmomanometer. Less often, but with increasing frequency, especially for major surgical procedures, a cannula is inserted into an artery, usually the radial artery at the wrist, and the blood pressure is measured directly from the artery during and after surgery. It is thus constantly available and, with the use of an appropriate *transducer*, it is possible to convert the pressure wave from the cannula into an electrical signal which can be constantly displayed on an *oscilloscope* screen and recorded on recording apparatus when required. The oscilloscope is usually also suitable for simultaneous display of the electrocardiogram.

Electrocardiogram

In the UK, ECG is being more frequently monitored during surgery and it is logical that this monitoring should be continued into the immediate postoperative period when appropriate (Fig. 3.1).

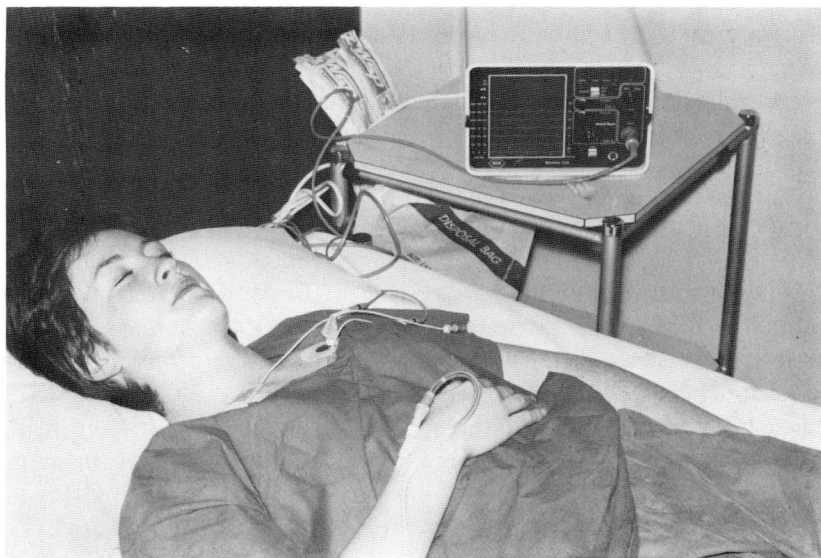

Fig. 3.1 *'Patient' with ECG monitor attached.*

A standard ECG for diagnostic purposes records from twelve different pairs of leads and thus twelve tracings showing different aspects of the electrical activity of the heart are available. Monitoring of the ECG, on the other hand, uses only one set of leads and the tracing available is therefore of less value than a full twelve-lead recording. Nevertheless, it is of value in showing the presence of changes in cardiac rhythm. If the nature of a rhythm disturbance is not clear from the monitor then a full twelve-lead ECG can help with diagnosis.

The other area where ECG monitoring may be of value is in the detection of *myocardial ischaemia*. Certain of the chest leads are of more value than others in demonstrating ischaemia and usually one of these is chosen for monitoring.

Most of the available ECG monitors in use today include a facility for displaying the heart rate, counted electronically from the electrocardiogram. It may be displayed as a digital read-out or by some other means. Most such monitors have a facility whereby, if the heart rate goes above or below a certain pre-selected range, an *alarm* will be triggered; the alarm may be available in the form of an audible bleep or a flashing light, or both.

Central venous pressure (CVP)

Central venous pressure is the pressure of the blood in the great veins inside the thorax—the superior and inferior venae cavae. It is an indication of the balance between the volume of blood in the circulation and the efficiency of the heart in pumping that blood around the circulation. It is measured using a manometer full of saline with the zero reference point at the midaxillary line at heart level. Certain manometers incorporate a spirit level which allows the zero point to be transferred accurately to a manometer scale graduated in centimetres above and below the zero mark (Fig. 3.2; Fig. 3.3). The pressure is measured through a catheter, the tip of which is positioned in the superior vena cava by inserting the catheter through a vein at the elbow or through one of the larger veins such as the internal (or occasionally external) jugular vein or the subclavian vein (Fig. 3.4). The normal CVP under these conditions is 5–10 cmH$_2$O. For convenience, the zero point is sometimes taken as the sternal angle, in which case

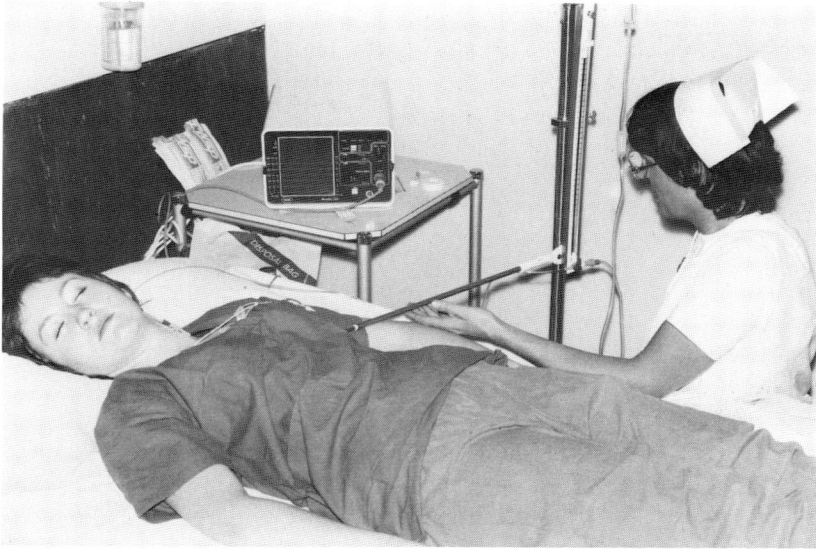

Fig 3.2 *Setting up the manometer to measure central venous pressure. A spirit level is used to identify accurately the zero level, which is at the mid-axillary line. This corresponds to the level of the right atrium of the heart.*

the normal pressure is 0–5 cmH$_2$O. During measurement, the level of the saline in the manometer will be seen to fluctuate by about 1 cm with the patient's respirations since the central venous pressure falls slightly during inspiration and rises again during expiration.

In order to measure CVP, the nurse must fill the open limb of the manometer with saline from the drip bottle or bag (*see* Fig. 3.3) by turning the three-way tap at the lower end of the manometer tube to the appropriate position. The three-way tap is then turned so that the manometer is connected through to the central venous catheter thus temporarily excluding the drip bottle and giving set. The level of fluid in the manometer tube will now fall until the hydrostatic pressure of the fluid in the tube equals the central venous pressure and can be read from the manometer tube in centimetres of water. Occasionally, if the patient is very hypovolaemic, the level will fall below zero and the CVP becomes negative, e.g. − 2 cmH$_2$O.

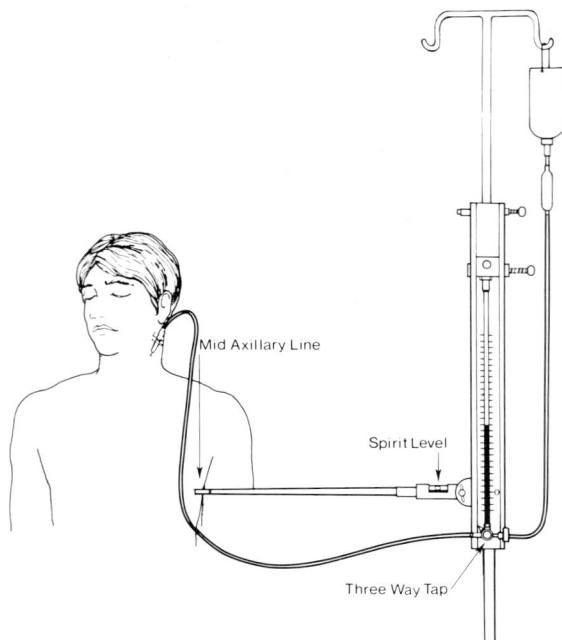

Fig. 3.3 *The central venous pressure manometer in use. The system is filled with saline from the drip. The catheter is entering the internal jugular vein in the neck. The spirit level is used to set up the manometer so that the zero level on the scale is level with the mid-axillary line. The three-way tap is used to fill the manometer and then to connect the manometer to the patient. When the level of saline in the manometer has settled, this indicates the level of the CVP (in cmH$_2$O).*

After making the reading of CVP, it is important for the nurse to remember to turn the three-way tap so that the drip is once again connected to the patient.

In the presence of good cardiac function a low CVP indicates a low blood volume. This is frequently due to blood loss during surgery or perhaps to other fluid loss from the body. CVP should be restored to normal by infusion of the appropriate fluid intravenously. This will of course be prescribed by a member of the medical staff.

A high CVP with good cardiac function indicates a degree of *over-transfusion* with fluid. If this becomes excessive there is a danger that

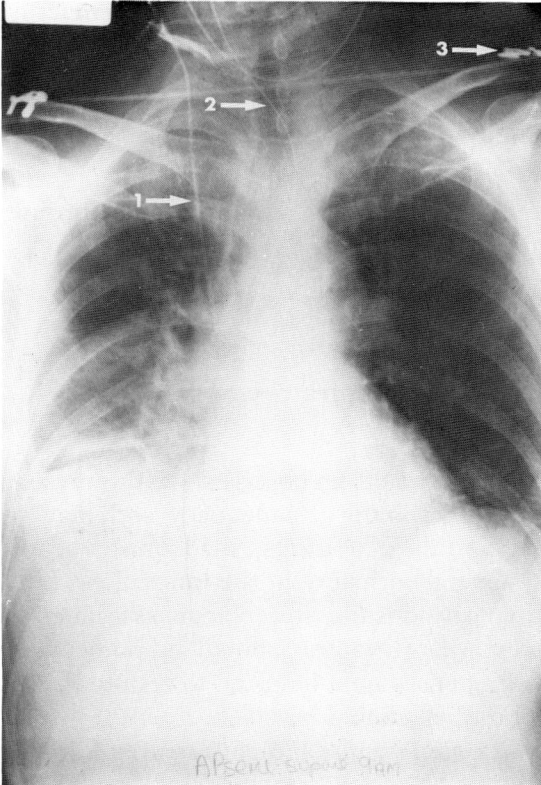

Fig. 3.4 *A chest x-ray showing a central venous catheter in the superior vena cava (1). The catheter has been inserted through the right internal jugular vein and is filled with contrast medium to make it easily visible. A nasogastric tube (2) and ECG electrodes (3) are also shown. N.B. There is an area of consolidation at the right lower lung zone.*

the lungs will become oedematous. Respiratory difficulty will then occur and cause *hypoxia* because oxygen cannot be transferred to blood as readily as usual when there is oedema of the lungs. In this situation, oxygen will have to be administered and an attempt to get rid of the excess fluid through the kidneys should be made by administering intravenously a rapidly-acting powerful diuretic such as frusemide. If these measures do not produce rapid improvement, it may be necessary to ventilate the patient's lungs artificially until improvement occurs.

In the presence of a normal blood volume, a high central venous pressure often indicates a degree of failure of cardiac function and drugs such as *digoxin* or other cardiac stimulants, for example the catecholamine *dopamine*, may be administered by intravenous infusion to improve this.

Respiratory System

The patient's colour should be observed for the presence of *cyanosis*. Cyanosis indicates respiratory inadequacy and may be due to respiratory depression due to drugs, inadequacy of the airway (*see* Chapter 4) or some abnormality in the lungs. Less often, cyanosis in the postoperative period is due to problems associated with the circulation. The presence of cyanosis should be immediately reported to the medical staff, steps should be taken to restore the patient's airway if need be, and oxygen should be given.

The patient's *respiratory rate* and pattern are of importance. Infants and small children have a normal respiratory rate in the region of 30–40 breaths per minute, whereas adults at rest breathe at a rate of about 10–20 breaths per minute. Slower rates are often associated with the administration of pain-relieving drugs such as morphine. Rapid shallow breathing may occur because of inadequately treated pain, especially after abdominal or thoracic surgery where deep breathing makes the pain worse. Rapid breathing may be present as a result of problems within the lungs and the patient, if awake, will usually complain of difficulty in breathing. A chest x-ray taken at this stage will often help to diagnose the cause. Persistence of the effects of *muscle relaxant* drugs given during anaesthesia may cause respiratory inadequacy. The use of a nerve stimulator to assess adequacy of neuromuscular transmission will help with the diagnosis of this condition.

Blood gases

The most readily available biochemical method of assessing adequacy of respiration is the estimation of blood gas partial pressures—that is the partial pressure of *oxygen* and *carbon dioxide* in the arterial blood. These give an indication of the adequacy of oxygenation of the blood and of the adequacy of carbon dioxide clearance by the lungs. A sample of blood from an artery is required and is usually taken from the radial artery at the wrist.

Oxygenation is indicated by the partial pressure of oxygen (Pao_2) in the arterial blood and is measured in kilopascals (kPa) or millimetres of mercury (mmHg). The normal level for a person with healthy lungs is 11.5–13 kPa or 85–100 mmHg. Elderly people may have slightly lower levels.

Reduction of the arterial oxygen partial pressure will occur in any condition where respiration is inadequate and the patient is breathing air. It will be elevated in the person who is breathing oxygen or oxygen-enriched air.

Normal function of the respiratory system is vital to the maintenance of the patient's *acid-base balance*. The normal products of tissue metabolism are acid in character and much of this acid is excreted from the lungs in the form of carbon dioxide. The partial pressure of carbon dioxide in the arterial blood therefore serves as an important indicator of respiratory function and tells us whether the patient is ventilating his lungs with an adequate amount of air. Normal partial pressure for arterial carbon dioxide ($Paco_2$) is 4.5–6 kPa or 35–45 mmHg and if the $Paco_2$ rises above this level it means that the lungs are being inadequately ventilated. Again this may be due to inadequacy of the airway, respiratory depression due to drugs, or some intrapulmonary abnormality.

When blood gases are checked, the pH of the patient's blood is also estimated, as is the base excess (BXS). The pH indicates whether the blood is *acidotic* or *alkalotic* (normal range 7.366–7.344) and the base excess tells if any pH abnormality is due to a metabolic type of acidosis or alkalosis. The normal range is between $+4$ and -4 mmol/l. A decrease from this range indicates metabolic acidosis and an increase indicates metabolic alkalosis.

Examples

1. A patient with partial *respiratory obstruction* breathing air might show the following results:

$$P_{ao_2} = 50 \text{ mmHg}; \ P_{aco_2} = 70 \text{ mmHg};$$
$$pH = 7.305; \ BXS = +2.5.$$

These results indicate poor oxygenation of the blood with diminished clearance of carbon dioxide. The retention of carbon dioxide has caused the pH to fall below normal—a respiratory acidosis. The metabolic component is within normal range (base excess normal).

2. The above patient is given 40% oxygen to breathe but his airway is still partially obstructed. After a few minutes of oxygen administration his blood gases are as follows:

$$P_{ao_2} = 110 \text{ mmHg}; \ P_{aco_2} = 80 \text{ mmHg};$$
$$pH = 7.300; \ BXS = +2.5.$$

Because of the increased oxygen supply, the patient's blood is now well oxygenated but his lungs are still poorly ventilated because the airway is still partially obstructed. He has therefore retained more carbon dioxide and become slightly more acidotic. The metabolic component is unaffected.

3. Finally, the patient's airway is cleared and he is still breathing 40% oxygen. After an hour or so his blood gases are:

$$P_{ao_2} = 160 \text{ mmHg}; \ P_{aco_2} = 45 \text{ mmHg};$$
$$pH = 7.367; \ BXS = +2.$$

There is now free access of the increased oxygen supply to the lungs and the oxygen level is therefore well above normal. Since the lungs can now ventilate adequately, the excess carbon dioxide is rapidly cleared bringing the P_{aco_2} back to normal, correcting the respiratory acidosis and bringing the pH back to normal.

4. A patient with chronic renal failure has undergone surgery and is now making an uneventful recovery breathing 40% oxygen. His gases are as follows:

$$Pao_2 = 150 \text{ mmHg}; Paco_2 = 30 \text{ mmHg};$$
$$pH = 7.290; BXS = -10.$$

The Pao_2 is elevated because he is breathing a higher than normal concentration of oxygen. The pH is low because the patient is acidotic. The base deficit of -10 indicates that the acidosis is metabolic in character and is due to the chronic renal failure. The carbon dioxide tension is low because the metabolic acidosis stimulates the respiratory centre to increase the minute volume of respiration thus reducing the $Paco_2$.

Chest x-ray

Frequently, where pulmonary dysfunction is suspected or thoracic surgery has been carried out, a chest x-ray will be requested in the recovery room. This will inevitably be a film taken with a mobile x-ray machine and will be taken with the patient lying flat on his back or propped up on pillows. The films are shot in the antero-posterior direction, which is the opposite direction to a film taken in the x-ray department. For these reasons, the film will be of different quality and therefore more difficult to interpret than the film taken in the x-ray department. However, it will show the presence of gross abnormalities such as an area of lung collapse or consolidation (Fig. 3.4) or a pneumothorax or haemothorax.

Renal Function

Patients who have had prolonged surgery (some operations in which the author has been involved recently have lasted more than 12 hours), patients who have had surgery associated with major blood loss and hypotension, and patients who have had poor renal function before their operations will require close observation of their renal function.

Urinary output

Assuming that the patient's blood volume and blood pressure are acceptable, the urinary output should be kept above a minimum of 30 ml/hour. This observation often requires that the patient's bladder should be catheterised and the nurse should observe and record the volume passed each hour. This is most easily done by allowing the urine to drain continuously into a graduated receptacle which can be emptied every hour (Fig. 3.5).

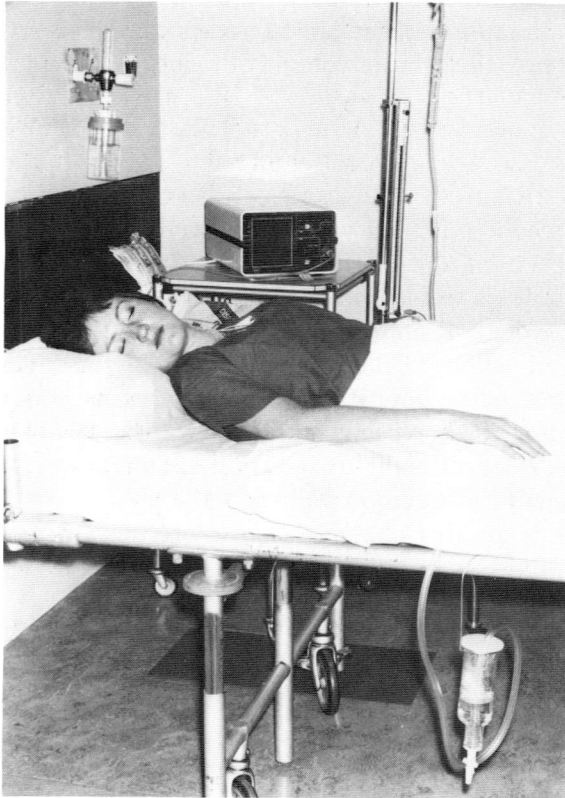

Fig. 3.5 *A urinary catheter is connected by tubing to a graduated vessel (a urimeter), thus allowing continuous measurement of urinary output.*

Low urine volume may result from low blood pressure or lowered blood volume or it may indicate failing renal function. If blood pressure is low this may also be due to low blood volume which will be indicated by a low central venous pressure. This will require correction by intravenous infusion of the appropriate fluid and will usually result in resumption of adequate urine volumes. If however the urine output does not respond to adequate fluid replacement then a diuretic such as frusemide or mannitol should be administered to increase urine flow.

Further checks on renal function will be required if low urine volumes persist. Comparison of urine to plasma osmolality gives an indication of the ability of the kidneys to concentrate urine. Biochemical estimations of plasma urea, creatinine and potassium should also be carried out but these are not likely to show meaningful changes in the very early hours of renal functional impairment. In renal failure, plasma urea, creatinine and potassium values will all tend to rise.

Sometimes the onset of renal failure will be marked by a high output of very dilute urine. This may continue for a time before the onset of oliguria. This 'high output' phase of renal failure should not be confused with the healthy kidney's response to an excessive load of intravenous fluid or to the normal response to administration of a rapidly-acting diuretic. Occasionally, certain forms of brain damage in the hypothalamic region can cause a reduction of antidiuretic hormone secretion from the pituitary gland. This will also have the effect of causing a large output of dilute urine. This latter condition is sometimes seen in patients after severe head injuries.

Haematological Monitoring

Patients who have had surgery associated with large volumes of blood loss and blood transfusion, and also patients who have had open heart surgery carried out with cardiopulmonary by-pass, will require to have certain haematological values estimated.

Haemoglobin level

This measurement gives an indication of the adequacy of replacement of blood loss and also, assuming that the blood volume replacement is adequate, indicates the amount of haemodilution which has taken place if the pre-operative haemoglobin level is known. Thus there is an estimate of the capacity of the blood to carry oxygen to the tissues since oxygen is attached to haemoglobin while it is transported in the blood.

Clotting factors

Blood stored in the blood bank has citrate solution added to it to prevent it from clotting during storage. Citrate has the effect of mopping up calcium ions in the blood which are necessary for the clotting process. Furthermore, many of the factors involved in the very complex process of blood clotting are unstable and tend very rapidly to become inactive in bank blood. Platelets are one of the cellular components of blood and are necessary in the clotting mechanism. They are also highly unstable and rapidly disintegrate in bank blood.

The absence of free calcium ions and the instability of other factors in the clotting chain mean that, when large volumes of bank blood are transfused, the patient's blood may fail to clot or may do so only very slowly. Thus, there is the possibility of postoperative haemorrhage.

The blood transfusion department can usually provide factors for replacement of those which are deficient, such as platelets which are removed from fresh donor blood. Since most of the other factors are unstable they cannot be prepared as individual components but are stabilised by freezing fresh donor plasma which is later unfrozen and prepared for transfusion as required.

If it is felt that the patient is in danger of having a clotting defect in the postoperative period, then a '*clotting screen*' should be requested. This necessitates certain samples of blood being sent to the haematology laboratory; the efficiency of the patient's clotting mechanism will be rapidly assessed and reported and a platelet count will be carried out at the same time. If necessary, platelets, fresh frozen plasma or other factors may be transfused.

Patients who have had heparin administered during the course of their operation (for example certain patients having vascular surgery) may require a check on their blood clotting postoperatively.

Biochemical Monitoring

Patients with certain illnesses, in addition to that for which they are being operated on, will require certain biochemical tests carried out postoperatively.

Diabetic patients

Patients with *diabetes mellitus*, especially the younger, more severe cases, may become unstable and develop swings in their blood sugar levels as a result of anaesthesia and surgery. Such patients therefore require checks on blood sugar postoperatively so that their insulin dosage and glucose intake may be adjusted. Insulin and glucose are usually given by intravenous infusion in the immediate postoperative period and this can cause the serum potassium level to fall. The potassium level will therefore also require to be checked and potassium given by intravenous infusion if necessary.

Patients who are known to have renal dysfunction will require to have specimens of blood removed for estimation of electrolyte levels (especially potassium) and blood urea within a few hours of operation.

Temperature Monitoring

The temperature of a patient may be recorded either as skin temperature or core temperature.

Skin temperature is usually recorded, as in usual ward procedure, by inserting a clinical thermometer into the axilla and reading it after a few minutes. This is satisfactory where only one or two temperature readings are anticipated during the patient's stay in the recovery room.

If, however, a prolonged stay in the recovery area is foreseen or if the patient's temperature is abnormal and will require frequent checking, skin temperature can be recorded by attaching a device called a thermocouple to the patient's skin, usually on the foot. A thermocouple is heat-sensitive and is connected by a wire to an electrical recording instrument which displays the temperature.

The skin temperature is influenced by two important factors. These are the environmental temperature and the amount of blood which is flowing through the skin capillaries at the time (i.e. the degree of vasodilatation or vasoconstriction in the skin).

The core temperature is measured by inserting a specially designed *thermocouple* into either the rectum or oesophagus. The normal reading is 37°C. (Skin temperature is usually one or two celsius degrees lower than core temperature.) Because the skin temperature is subject to the influences mentioned above, the core temperature usually gives a more meaningful indication of the true body temperature. For example, if a person has been exposed to cold for some time, his skin temperature may be as low as 31°C, but at the same time his core temperature may be nearly normal, for example, 36.5°C. The skin temperature will be low because of heat loss from the skin to the cold environment, and also because the sympathetic nervous system will cause a reduction of the blood flow to the cold skin in order to preserve heat to maintain the core temperature at a normal or near normal level. The importance of maintaining the core temperature at a normal level is so that the important organs such as the heart, brain, liver and kidneys can continue to function normally as the enzymes involved in the metabolism of body organs and tissues function most efficiently at about 37°C.

Effect of anaesthesia and surgery on body temperature

Normally the core temperature is maintained at 37°C because the heat produced by the body is balanced by the heat lost. Heat is produced by metabolism of the vital organs and, in addition, by the activity of muscles. The muscles of respiration are constantly in use and therefore produce heat at all times but other muscles vary in their heat production according to their activity.

Heat is lost from the body surface; the amount of heat lost depends on the amount of insulating clothing and on the environmental temperature. Moisture is constantly being vapourised from the skin surface as both sensible and insensible perspiration. The evaporation of perspiration requires latent heat, most of which comes from the skin.

Heat is also lost from the respiratory tract since air inhaled at environmental temperature is heated and exhaled at body temperature.

During anaesthesia, the metabolism of the vital organs continues but muscle activity, often even that of the respiratory muscles, is abolished and so only basal heat production by vital organs occurs. Heat loss, however, takes place in the normal way from the skin, the amount depending on the insulation provided by the surgical drapes and on the theatre temperature. Furthermore, the normal mechanism of vasoconstriction in response to heat loss may be reduced or abolished by certain anaesthetic drugs and so heat loss may occur at a faster rate than usual. Heat loss will also continue from the respiratory tract whether the patient is breathing spontaneously or is artificially ventilated during his operation since the gases which he is breathing will be at room temperature.

It is obvious from the above that the patient's temperature will tend to fall during his operation because heat production is less than normal and heat loss is likely to be higher than normal. If the surgery is prolonged and especially if large areas of tissue are exposed by major surgery, the temperature drop may be considerable.

Small children tend to lose heat more rapidly than adults because weight for weight they have a larger skin surface area.

If conditions are foreseen where there will be a large heat loss during surgery, steps should be taken to limit this as much as possible so that the patient's temperature will be kept as near normal as possible. The steps to be taken will include raising the temperature of the theatre and applying extra surgical drapes to the patient. Other measures which will be helpful in limiting heat loss are warming of transfused blood and other fluids and also the warming of gases to be breathed by the patient. Both of these measures are achieved by using specially designed devices.

Hypothermia

Despite all the above measures, the patient may be cold when he arrives in the recovery room; if an initial check on the skin tempertaure confirms this, skin and core temperature should be recorded until rewarming has occurred. This will involve applying a skin thermocouple to a foot and inserting a rectal thermocouple into the rectum.

As indicated earlier, the temperature difference between these two sites may be quite marked and the extent to which the skin temperature is lower than the rectal temperature will indicate the degree of skin vasoconstriction which has occurred in response to the falling temperature. Steps similar to those taken to maintain the patient's temperature in theatre will be required in the recovery room and, as the patient recovers from the anaesthesia thus getting rid of the anaesthetic drugs and regaining muscle activity, his temperature will begin to return towards normal and his skin temperature will again begin to approximate to his core temperature. Frequently, patients will be seen to shiver. This causes the temperature to rise fairly rapidly.

It is rarely necessary to take steps to warm the patient actively, i.e. applying warming devices such as an electric blanket. If the patient's temperature should continue to fall, however, and especially if the core temperature approaches 30°C, active warming measures should be started. If the core temperature falls below 30°C there is a danger that cardiac arrhythmias, especially ventricular fibrillation, may occur.

If active warming is necessary, great care must be taken that no warming device reaches a temperature greater than 37°C and that no area of the patient's skin is in contact with a warm area for more than a few minutes; otherwise, burning of the skin may occur.

Elevated temperature

It is rare for a patient with a raised temperature to have elective surgery carried out. Not infrequently, however, emergency surgery may be required for a patient with pyrexia due to a surgically treatable infection such as an abscess. In this case, the temperature will be elevated postoperatively and appropriate antibiotic drugs should be prescribed. Occasionally tepid sponging may be indicated as a means of cooling the patient.

Sometimes the steps taken in theatre to prevent the patient's temperature from falling may be so successful that the tempertaure may actually rise. It is unusual for the temperature to rise above 38°C from this cause and the temperature soon self-corrects after the operation.

Malignant hyperpyrexia

This is a very rare but extremely serious anaesthetic-related condition which results in a rapid rise in the patient's temperature during or immediately following anaesthesia. It is genetically determined and causes an abnormal response of the patients's muscles to certain anaesthetic drugs, especially suxamethonium (a short-acting depolarising muscle relaxant) and halothane (an inhalational agent), but other drugs have also been shown to trigger the condition.

When malignant hyperpyrexia is diagnosed, any drug known to be a trigger agent should be discontinued. Active cooling should be started and the surgery and anaesthesia should be terminated as soon as possible. Active cooling will be required in the recovery area and should take the form of ice packs and wet sheets on the patient's skin, fans blowing on the patient, and infusion of cold intravenous fluids. The drug Dantrolene is thought to be helpful in controlling the disordered metabolism of the muscles and should be given as soon as possible by intravenous infusion. Because of the high temperature and extremely high rate of metabolism in the muscle tissue, the patient's oxygen requirement and usage will be much greater than normal and oxygen should be given in as high a concentration as possible. For the same reason his rate of carbon dioxide production will be much higher than normal and, if breathing spontaneously, his rate of breathing will be rapid and deep, so that his minute volume will be very large. If he is being artificially ventilated, the settings of the ventilator will probably have to be such as to give maximum minute volume. In addition, there is always a degree of metabolic acidosis which will require treatment with sodium bicarbonate solution given intravenously. Unless malignant hyperpyrexia is diagnosed quickly after its onset and treated rapidly and very actively, it will be fatal.

When treatment is successful, the temperature begins to fall fairly rapidly but it has been known to start rising again after a short time and so the patient must remain in recovery or intensive care with close observation of temperature for at least 12 hours.

CHAPTER 4

The Airway

The airway is the passage by which air moves from the surrounding atmosphere into and out of the lungs. It consists of the mouth and nasal passages, the pharynx, larynx, trachea and bronchi.

Attention to the airway is one of the most important aspects of patient care in the immediate postoperative period. If a patient does not have a clear airway, he will be unable to breathe freely and, as a result, his life will be in danger.

It is the responsibility of the anaesthetist to ascertain that the patient has a clear airway before handing him over to the care of the recovery room staff.

Most patients who are unconscious will require some form of airway support. The airway becomes blocked because the tongue tends to fall back against the palate and posterior pharyngeal wall, thus making it difficult for air to pass from the nose or mouth into the larynx. This is most likely to happen when the patient is lying on his back (Fig. 4.1). A minor form of this kind of airway obstruction is seen in persons who snore when they are asleep. The snoring noise is due to vibration of the tongue or palate as the air passes through the naso-oral air passage.

Saliva and mucus from the mouth, and blood when there has been surgery in the nose, mouth or throat, may also be responsible for causing a certain degree of respiratory obstruction. If saliva, mucus or blood find their way into the larynx, they may cause laryngeal spasm—that is a complete or partial reflex closure of the larynx to the passage of air.

All patients will have a certain quantity of gastric secretions in their stomach. Patients who have been operated on under emergency con-

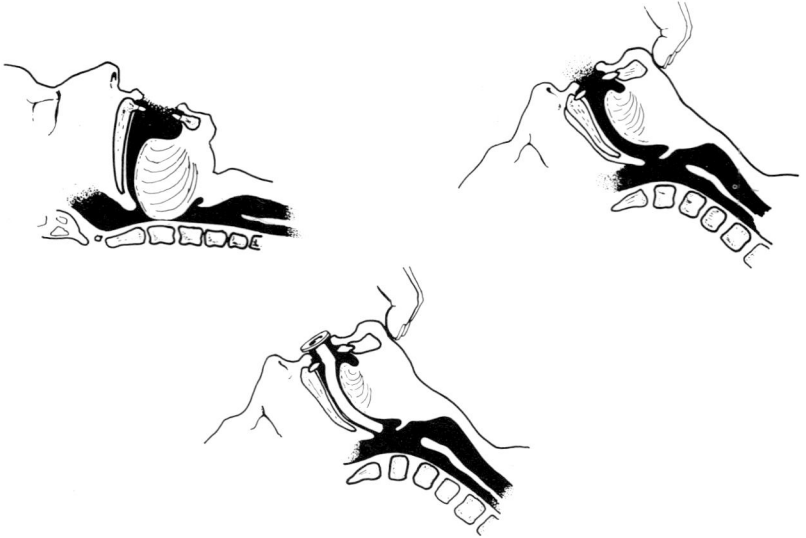

Fig. 4.1 *Upper left: how the airway may be obstructed by the tongue falling back against the posterior wall of the pharynx in the unconscious patient.*
Upper right: how the tongue is pulled forward when the chin is supported. Sometimes this is not enough to clear the airway properly and an artificial airway is required as shown in the diagram below.

ditions may have taken food or drink shortly before operation and have a fairly large gastric content. This may be regurgitated or vomited during the recovery phase and will be a potentially serious cause of respiratory obstruction. Furthermore, gastric contents are often highly acidic in character and, if inhaled into the lungs, can produce a serious and life-threatening form of chemical damage to the lungs (Mendelsson's syndrome).

Certain faciomaxillary operations pose major potential airway problems, for example some patients have their jaws wired together at the end of their operation and therefore the only access to the airway is through the nose.

Recognition of Respiratory Obstruction

To recognise the presence of respiratory obstruction it is important to know what the normal respiratory pattern in a sleeping person looks and sounds like. During quiet breathing when the airway is clear, there is little sound from the passage of air in and out of the mouth and nose and indeed it may be necessary to put one's ear close to the patient's face to hear any sound at all. This is especially true in children who normally have a small tidal volume. The pattern of movement of the chest and abdomen is important. Normally the chest and abdomen move in unison so that the chest wall and abdominal wall rise and fall together as the patient breathes in and out. There is virtually no visible movement of the larynx or trachea.

In contrast to this picture of calm, obstruction-free breathing, the patient who has respiratory obstruction exhibits certain features which differ considerably.

There may be clearly audible respiratory sounds. A snoring sound is common and always indicates a certain degree of respiratory obstruction. It should not be tolerated in the patient who is recovering from anaesthesia. Patients who have partial laryngeal occlusion due to laryngeal spasm produce laryngeal stridor which is a high-pitched 'crowing' sound during inspiration. The presence of fluid (saliva, mucus, blood or gastric contents) in the mouth and pharynx produces a gurgling or bubbling sound and may cause the patient to cough or hold his breath.

The respiratory pattern is abnormal when there is respiratory obstruction. The normal smooth rise and fall of chest and abdomen is replaced by a much more jerky type of pattern where, during inspiration, the abdomen is pushed outwards and the upper part of the chest wall is pulled inwards thus giving rise to a 'see-saw' type of pattern. In severe degrees of respiratory obstruction there will be 'tracheal tug' which results in the larynx (Adam's apple) being pulled downwards about a centimetre during inspiration and sliding back upwards during expiration. The alae nasae may also dilate during inspiration. The accessory respiratory muscles, e.g. the sternomastoid, will be seen to contract strongly during inspiration.

These changes in the respiratory pattern are due to the increased muscular efforts which the patient makes in an effort to overcome the obstruction to the passage of air, and the amount of disturbance to the normal pattern will depend on the degree of obstruction present.

The Consequences of Airway Obstruction

When the airway is totally obstructed, no air at all can reach the lungs and this, if not corrected, will rapidly lead to death from lack of oxygen.

When there is partial blockage of the airway, some air, but less than necessary, will reach the lungs. Therefore there will be *hypoxia*, the degree of which will depend on the severity of obstruction. If the patient is breathing room air this will result in cyanosis. If the patient is breathing oxygen, however, there may not be cyanosis since the lungs may then receive enough oxygen to fully oxygenate the blood. Nevertheless, if there is evidence of airway obstruction, this must be corrected since the total amount of air which reaches the lungs will still be less than is necessary to remove the carbon dioxide from the blood. In other words, the lungs are inadequately ventilated and respiratory acidosis will occur. A raised carbon dioxide level in the blood (respiratory acidosis) is a very powerful stimulus to respiration and causes the patient to make even greater respiratory efforts. This has the effect of making the respiratory pattern appear more grossly abnormal and causes the muscles of respiration to work harder. They will therefore require more oxygen than in the resting patient with a clear airway and hence the onset of hypoxia will be more likely.

Thus respiratory obstruction gives rise to hypoxia and respiratory acidosis in the patient who is breathing air. The administration of oxygen may temporarily correct the hypoxia but it will not correct the respiratory acidosis and so oxygen should only be used as a means of preventing or overcoming hypoxia. A clear airway must be re-established to allow good lung ventilation, to clear excess carbon dioxide from the blood, and to correct respiratory acidosis (*see* Ch. 3).

Because of the large respiratory muscular effort that is made during obstructed breathing, the negative pressure generated within the chest during inspiration will be much greater than normal. If this is allowed to continue it is believed that it can have the effect of encouraging an excessive amount of fluid to accumulate in the lungs (*pulmonary oedema*). If this should occur, hypoxia will become even more severe.

Prevention and Correction of Airway Obstruction

Positioning of the patient

Many potential airway problems can be prevented by correct position-ing of the patient during recovery from anaesthesia. Where the sur-gery permits it, the patient should be nursed on his side (Fig. 4.2).

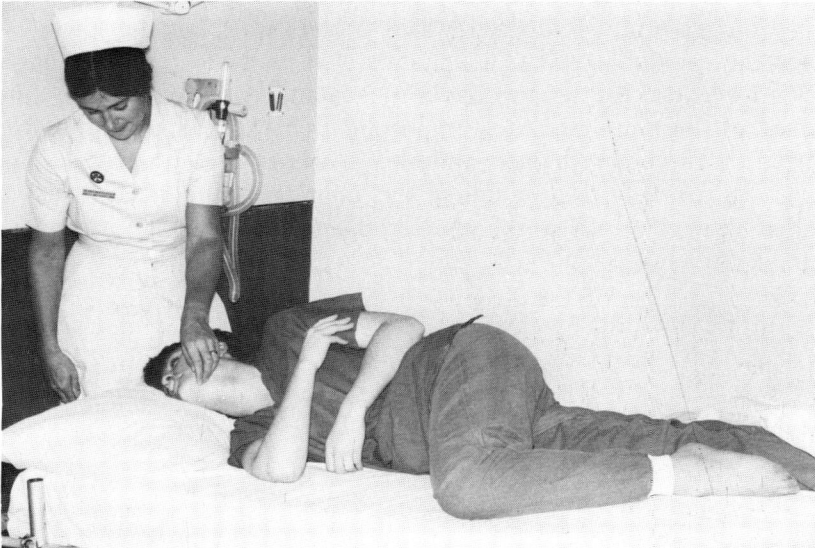

Fig. 4.2 *Subject in the right lateral position with the nurse holding the chin upward and forward so that the airway remains clear. Note that the nurse's fingers are applied to the mandible and not to the soft tissues under the chin. The legs are pos-itioned so that the 'patient' will not roll on to her face and the arms are placed in a 'comfortable' position to avoid damage to joints and pressure on nerves and blood vessels.*

The lateral position is helpful because it encourages the tongue to fall away from the pharynx and palate and this helps to keep the airway clear. Furthermore, if there has been surgery in the mouth, nose or throat (for example, tonsillectomy), blood will be encouraged to run out of the nose or mouth rather than backwards towards the larynx.

This is especially so if, as well as keeping the patient in the lateral position, the trolley is tilted a few degrees head downwards. This position is also valuable if the patient is suspected of having a full stomach, as vomited or regurgitated gastric contents will also tend to run out of the mouth.

The position of the head is important. To maintain the best position for keeping the airway open, the neck should be flexed forward and the head extended. This is sometimes referred to as the 'sniffing the morning air' position. The head should be held in this position by firmly but carefully pulling upwards and forward on the lower jaw bone (the mandible) (Fig. 4.3). This also tends to pull the tongue forward because the tongue has a muscular attachment to the inner surface of the mandible. It is important that the pressure should be exerted on the bone of the mandible. If it is exerted by pressing upwards on the soft tissues under the chin then the tongue will be pushed upwards against the roof of the mouth and the air passage through the mouth will be occluded.

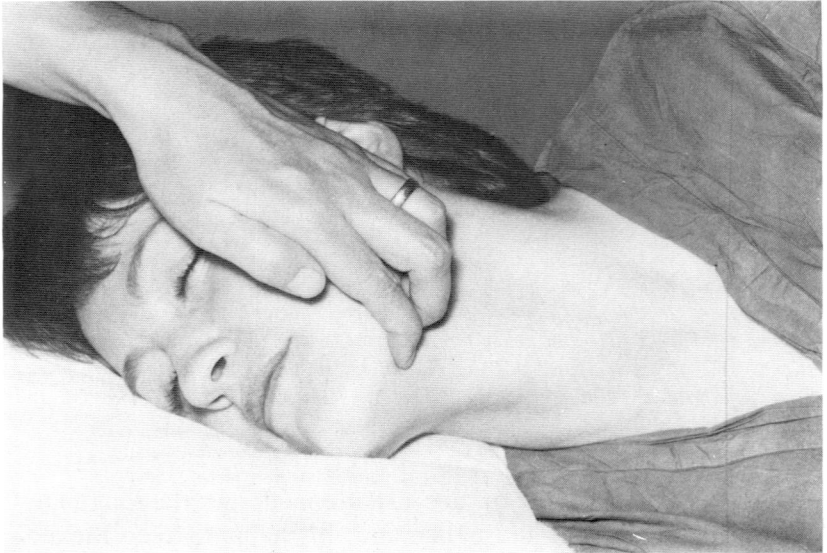

Fig. 4.3 *Close-up showing chin held correctly by firmly holding the mandible upwards and forward. It is important to ensure that the eyes are closed so that the cornea cannot be accidentally damaged by rubbing against the pillow.*

The use of artificial airways

Despite correct positioning of the patient, there are many instances where it remains difficult to maintain a clear airway in the unconscious patient. This is likely to happen, for example, in obese patients with large tongues, in elderly, edentulous patients where cheeks and lips tend to collapse inwards and obstruct the airway, and in certain patients who have had intra-oral operations because of swelling of the tongue and other tissues inside the mouth. Children who have enlarged tonsils and adenoids can also produce airway difficulties.

Many of the above types of patients can have their airway problems alleviated by the use of an artificial airway and, indeed, most of them will have an artificial airway in place when they come to the recovery area from theatre. This will have been inserted by the anaesthetist during anaesthesia.

The commonest type of artificial airway in present day use is the Guedel oropharyngeal airway (Fig. 4.4; Fig. 4.5). This is simply a

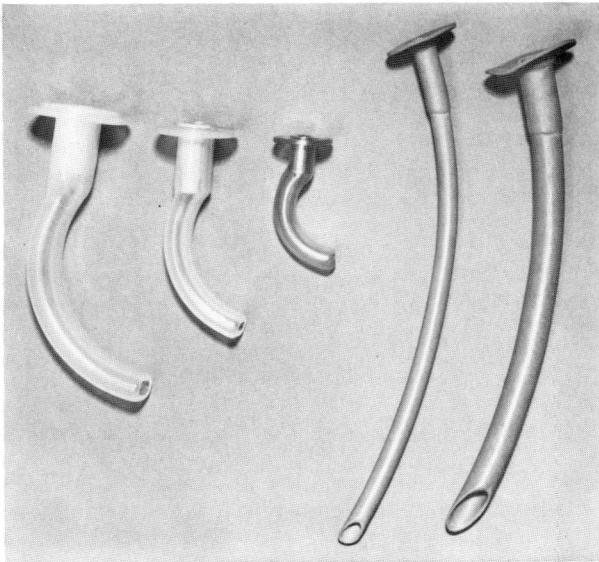

Fig. 4.4 *Left: three sizes of Guedel oropharyngeal airways. The curved nature of the tube is evident, and the flange at the upper (outer) end. The reinforced area behind the flange is also shown. Right: two nasopharyngeal airways.*

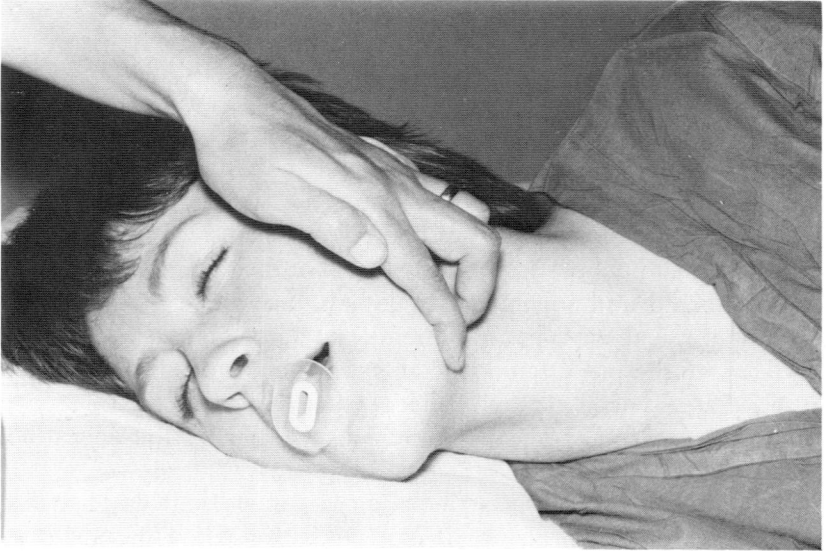

Fig. 4.5 *An oropharyngeal airway in place. The part between the teeth is reinforced to prevent obstruction by biting.*

flattened tube made of rubber or plastic, curved so as to pass through the mouth and over the back of the tongue. The outer end has a flange which rests against the lips and prevents it from slipping too far back. The part immediately behind the flange is strengthened so that, if the patient should bite on it as he recovers, it will not be occluded. The length of the Guedel airway is such that the inner end lies in the pharynx just above the larynx (*see* Fig. 4.1) and various sizes, numbered 1 to 4, are available to suit different sizes of patients. A size 2 or 3 is suitable for most women and a size 3 of 4 for most men.

It has been stated earlier that most of the patients who require an artificial airway will already have it in place on admission to the recovery room. Sometimes, however, an airway difficulty will develop during recovery and require the insertion of an artificial airway at that stage. It may be possible to insert a Guedel airway into the mouth but often the patient may have recovered to such an extent that he will not retain an oral airway (he has become 'too light') or perhaps the teeth may be clenched and it is impossible to insert an oral airway. In such cases the use of a nasopharyngeal airway should be considered.

A *nasopharyngeal airway* (Fig. 4.4) is simply a curved tube which can be passed through the nose. It has a flange at the outer end (Fig. 4.6). It is often a very helpful means of dealing with the obstructed air passage. It should be inserted gently since the nasal mucous membrane is easily damaged and bleeds readily. For this reason the nasopharyngeal airway is made of soft rubber. Many patients have a deviated nasal septum and the nasal airway will pass more easily through one nostril than the other. It is important to remember that, once the external opening of the nose has been entered, the nasal passage goes directly backwards and not upwards, and therefore the nasal airway should be directed backwards. A full range of sizes of

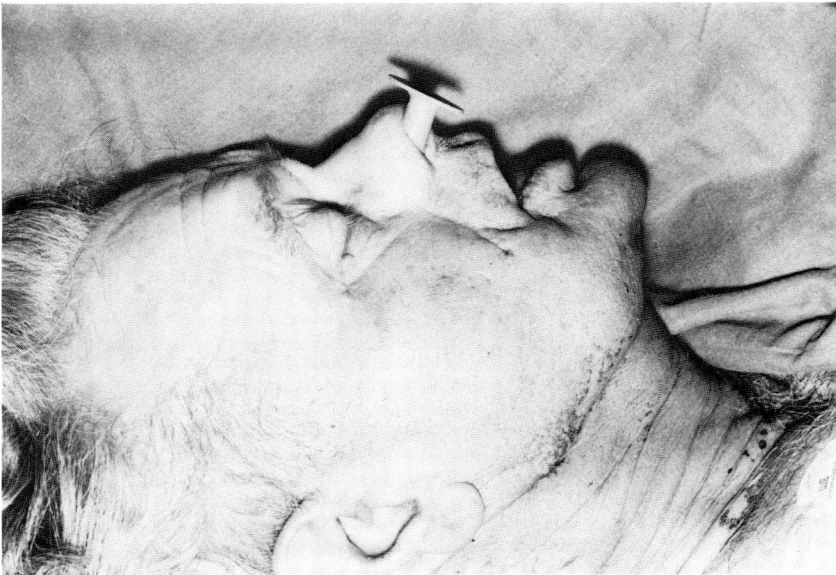

Fig. 4.6 *A nasopharyngeal airway used to help maintain a clear air passage in a patient who has undergone minor intra-oral surgery and in whom an oral airway would be unsuitable.*

nasal airways is available. In the absence of a specially designed nasopharyngeal airway, a shortened endotracheal tube can be used.

As the patient recovers or 'becomes lighter' he will often tend to eject an oral airway by coughing or pushing it out with his tongue. Some will wake up with the airway still in place and be unaware of its presence until they try to speak. They will then eject it or the nurse may remove it. A nasopharyngeal airway will have to be removed by the nurse when the patient has recovered sufficiently.

Occasionally it will be difficult to restore a patient's airway even with the use of an oral or nasal airway. This may occur as a result of a severe episode of *laryngeal spasm*. In such a case the help of the medical staff should be immediately summoned since, very occasionally, it may be necessary to insert a tracheal tube into the patient's trachea and this is usually undertaken by the anaesthetist. To allow intubation, the patient may be turned onto his back but the left lateral position is also acceptable for this procedure. The McIntosh *laryngoscope* (Fig. 4.7), which is the instrument most commonly used to visualise the larynx for intubation, is designed so that the tongue is pushed over to the left side of the mouth, making it much more awkward to use if the patient were in the right lateral position when the tongue would naturally fall towards the right side of the mouth. A cuffed *tracheal tube* is usually used (Fig. 4.7).

Once intubated, the patient's airway will be restored and the tube can be left in place until the patient has recovered.

Secretions from the respiratory tract may be sucked out by passing a catheter through the tracheal tube.

Severe postoperative airway difficulties can be predicted in certain patients. Among these are patients who have had reconstructive plastic procedures around the mouth and nose, those who have had bony surgery in the faciomaxillary area and may have their jaws wired together, and those who have difficulty flexing their necks or extending their heads. The latter group includes patients with severe burn scars, or previous surgery in the neck region, and those with rheumatoid arthritis of the cervical spine.

Such patients will have had tracheal intubation during anaesthesia and it is likely that the tracheal tube will be left in place until the patient is well recovered and able to maintain an airway indepen-

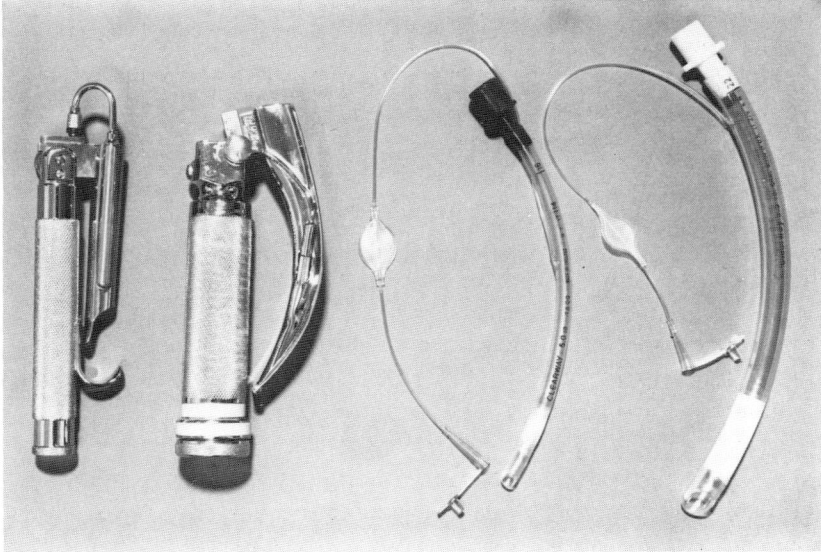

Fig. 4.7 *Left: a straight bladed laryngoscope of suitable size for use in infants and small children. Alongside is an adult-sized, curved bladed (McIntosh) laryngoscope. In use, the laryngoscope is unfolded so that the blade is at right angles to the handle. This makes an electrical contact which lights a bulb near the tip of the blade so that intubation of the trachea is made easier. The power to light the bulb is supplied by batteries in the handle. Right: two sizes of cuffed tracheal tubes. When a tube is in place, the fine tube attached to the main tube is used to inflate the cuff which is the white area at the lower end of the main tube. The cuff is inflated with air from a syringe.*

dently (Fig. 4.8). The tracheal tube in many of these cases will be passed through the nose (Fig. 4.9). This is advantageous for the recovery room staff since a nasotracheal tube is usually tolerated much more readily by the recovering patient than an orotracheal tube and will therefore be retained longer before the patient starts to cough and reject the tube.

If it is anticipated that an airway difficulty will persist after recovery from anaesthesia, a tracheostomy should be performed at the time of the operation (Fig. 4.10). Although a tracheal tube is the most effective means of providing an artificial airway, it is not an absolute

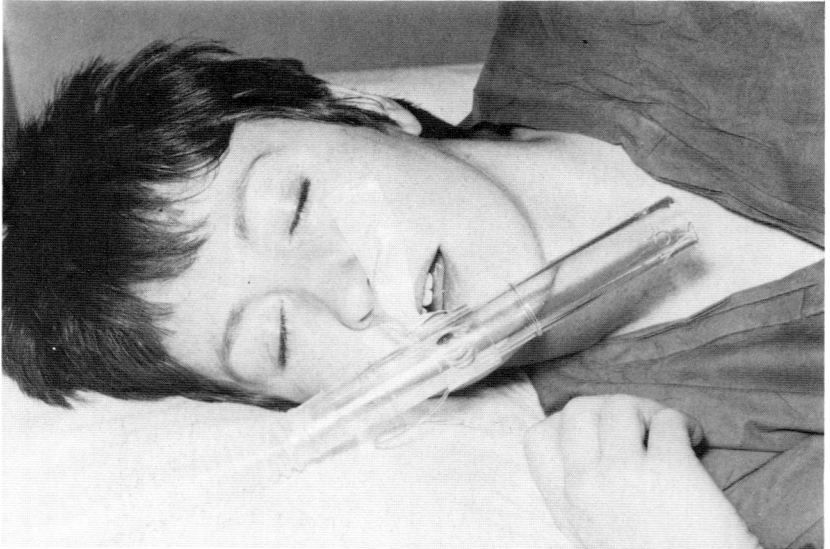

Fig. 4.8 *An orotracheal tube left in place during recovery. Humidified oxygen-enriched air is suppled to the 'patient' through the corrugated tubing.*

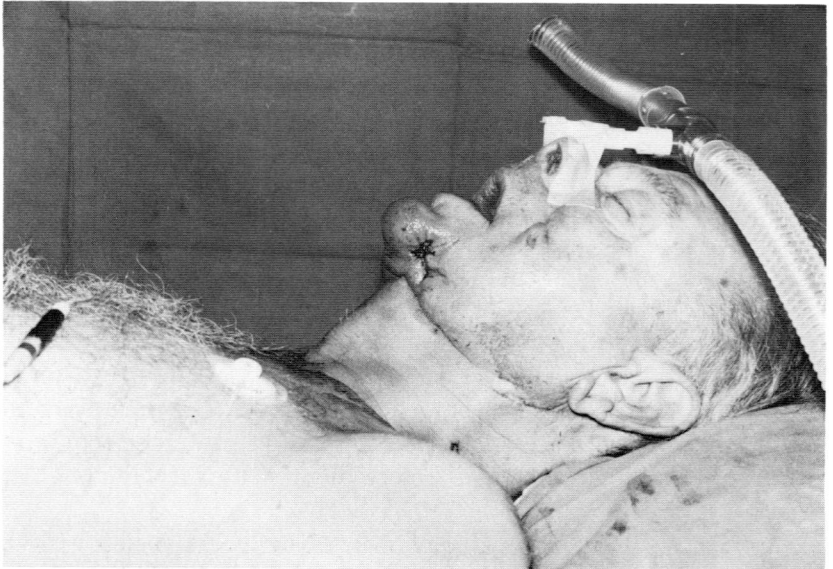

Fig. 4.9 *A patient with a nasotracheal tube in place following major intra-oral surgery. Oxygen is supplied through the wide-bore corrugated tube passing across the patient's forehead.*

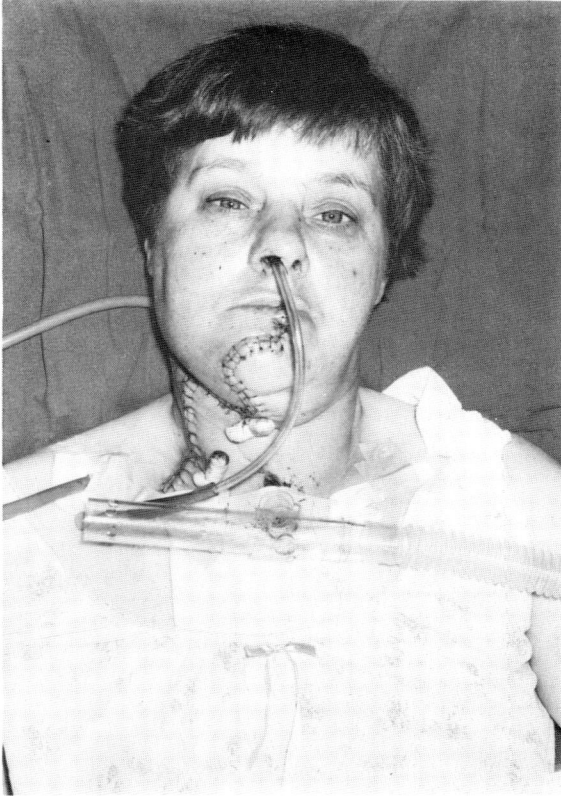

Fig. 4.10 *This patient has undergone extensive surgery involving the floor of the mouth, tongue, mandible and neck. Because of swelling and distortion of the tissues inside the mouth which would cause obstruction to breathing, the patient is breathing humidified air through a tracheostomy. The corrugated tubing carrying the humidified air is attached to the tracheostomy tube by a 'T' piece. The tracheostomy tube will be removed when the swelling subsides and healing is progressing satisfactorily. The patient will be unable to swallow for some time after her operation and so a nasogastric tube has also been inserted. She can now receive fluids and a liquidised diet through the nasogastric tube.*

guarantee of a clear air passage since the tube can become blocked by mucus or blood clot. It is important therefore that the patient's respiratory pattern should still be carefully observed when a tracheal tube is in place or when a tracheostomy has been done.

The use of suction

An efficient source of suction must always be provided in the recovery area. It will be required for the removal of secretions, blood or gastric contents from the mouth, nose and throat, and may also be required for applying suction to surgical drains.

As previously pointed out, patients who have had operations in the nose, mouth or throat should be nursed in the lateral position with a slight head-down tilt to encourage blood to drain away from the larynx. Gentle suction with a soft rubber catheter should be applied initially via the mouth and nose to remove any blood which may have collected during transport to the recovery area. If an oral or nasal airway or tracheal tube is in place, a sterile catheter may be passed through the airway or alongside the oral airway or tube (Fig. 4.11).

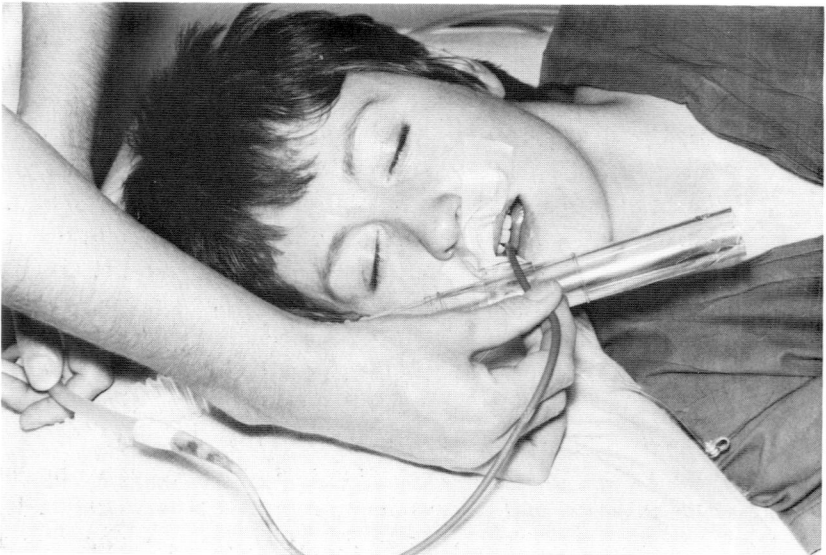

Fig. 4.11 *A nurse applies suction to remove secretions from the mouth. A flexible catheter is passed to the back of the pharynx alongside the tracheal tube. If necessary, a fresh sterile catheter can be passed through the tracheal tube to suck out secretions from the bronchial tree.*

Insertion of the catheter should be gentle so that raw surfaces, such as a tonsil bed after tonsillectomy, will not be stimulated to produce further bleeding. If bleeding is continuous, a catheter may be passed through the nose into the pharynx and left with suction attached until the bleeding stops.

Many patients will have been given an anticholinergic drug such as atropine or hyoscine as part of their premedication and this will reduce the volume of secretions produced by the salivary glands and hence no suction will be necessary. If however secretions can be seen or heard in the mouth or pharynx, suction should be applied, as above, for their removal.

If a patient vomits or regurgitates stomach contents, the trolley should be immediately tilted head downwards and vigorous suction applied to the pharynx through the mouth or nose. In this case, a catheter with as wide a bore as possible should be used. Medical help should be summoned because it will be preferable for the pharynx to be sucked out under direct vision using a laryngoscope (Fig. 4.12). A rigid type of suction attachment, such as the Yankauer type of sucker, is preferable in this situation since it can be directed, under vision, to any area of the pharynx to remove vomited material.

If the patient is thought to have inhaled vomit, tracheal intubation will be required to suck out as much as possible of the inhaled material from the trachea and bronchi and possibly also to carry out *bronchial lavage*. Bronchial lavage is a procedure where small quantities (up to 20 ml in an adult) of physiological saline (0.9% sodium chloride solution) are injected into the bronchial tree through a fine catheter which is passed through the tracheal tube. Each injection of saline is sucked back using a suction catheter through the tracheal tube and it is hoped that the inhaled material will be removed with or diluted by the saline and thus be less irritating to the respiratory tract.

When a tracheal tube is in place, and suction is required through the tube, the diameter of the catheter used for suction must be less than half of that of the tracheal tube, otherwise it is possible that an excessively high amount of negative pressure will be applied to the respiratory tract and may cause acute collapse of parts of the lungs. The smaller the tracheal tube, the more important is this point and hence it is most important in small children and infants.

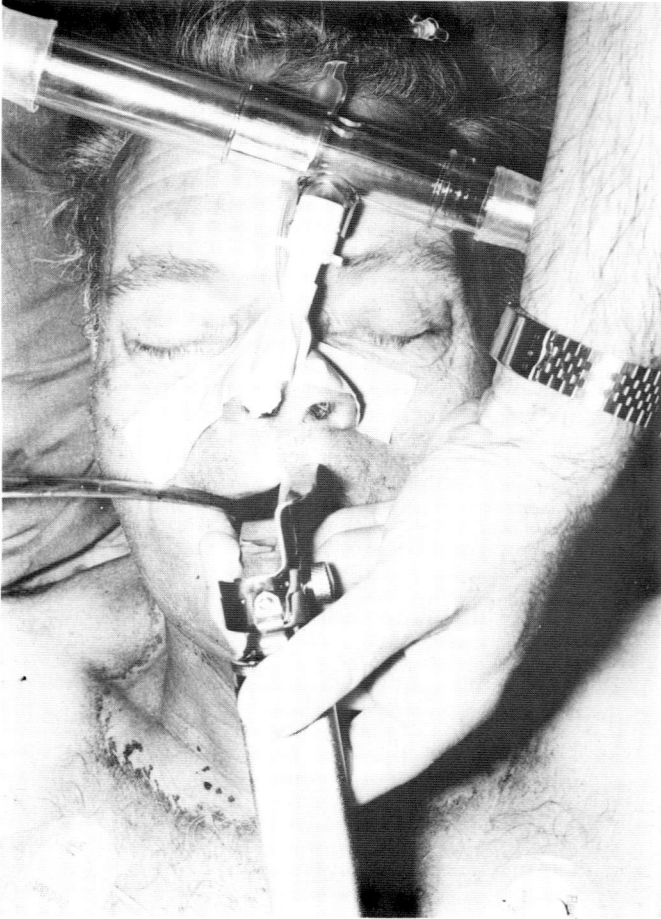

Fig 4.12 *Under direct vision, blood is sucked out from a patient's mouth and throat following intra-oral surgery. A laryngoscope and a rigid suction nozzle are used in these circumstances. This patient has a nasotracheal tube in place.*

CHAPTER 5

Pain Relief

The relief of pain, especially pain occurring in the postoperative period, is often one of the problems least effectively dealt with, despite the fact that effective methods are available for relieving pain. There are several reasons for this, one of the most important of which is that the appreciation of pain varies very much from patient to patient and an operation which may cause one patient only some discomfort may cause another to experience a significant degree of pain. Furthermore, pain-relieving drugs tend to be administered in standard doses and so some patients will receive an inadequate dose relative to their body weight and others may receive more than necessary to make them comfortable.

Methods of giving pain relief

A number of methods for relieving pain are available. These are listed as follows:
1. Intermittent injections of analgesic drugs.
2. Continuous intravenous infusion of analgesic drugs.
3. Inhalation analgesia.
4. Nerve blocks.
5. Regional blocks.
6. Oral analgesics.

Intermittent Injections of Analgesic Drugs

This is the commonest method of administering analgesic drugs in the immediate postoperative period but it is also the method least likely to produce satisfactory relief of pain.

Drugs to be given by intermittent injections are often prescribed on an 'as required' basis with a minimum time between injections stated, e.g. '4 hourly, as required', thus leaving the timing of the injections broadly to the judgement of the nursing staff. It also requires the patient to indicate to the nurse that his pain is returning or becoming more severe as the effect of each dose of analgesia wears off. Thus, the pain relief is intermittent and the pain returns between doses of the drug.

Subcutaneous injections should not be used since absorption of the drug is fairly slow from the subcutaneous area. The drug should be given intramuscularly or preferably intravenously. If the intravenous route is used, the drugs will have to be administered by a doctor. Drugs to be given intravenously should be diluted; for example, morphine is administered intramuscularly in a concentration of 10 mg/ml of solution, but for intravenous use it should be diluted with sterile water to give a concentration of 1 mg/ml. This is then given to the patient in small increments of 1 or 2 mg until a satisfactory level of analgesia is obtained. Thereafter, similar small doses are given as required.

Drugs used for intermittent injection

These are mainly of the narcotic analgesic type such as morphine, papaveretum and pethidine. Morphine, as well as being a potent analgesic drug, has a euphoric effect which is helpful in allaying the patient's anxiety and it also makes the patient sleepy. Other drugs such as buprenorphine or pentazocine may be used.

Continuous Intravenous Infusion of Analgesic Drugs

This is a much more satisfactory method of producing pain relief than the use of intermittent injections.

The intravenous infusion may be started after a satisfactory level of analgesia has been obtained by giving small increments intravenously, or it may be started immediately on admission to the recovery room so that an effect continuous with any narcotic analgesics given during anaesthesia may be maintained. The drug to be used has to be diluted and must be administered from an infusion pump (Fig. 5.1), which is a device specially designed to accept the syringe containing the diluted drug and inject the drug at a pre-set slow rate, for example 1–6 mg/hour for morphine. The major advantage of this method is that it is continuous and, once established,

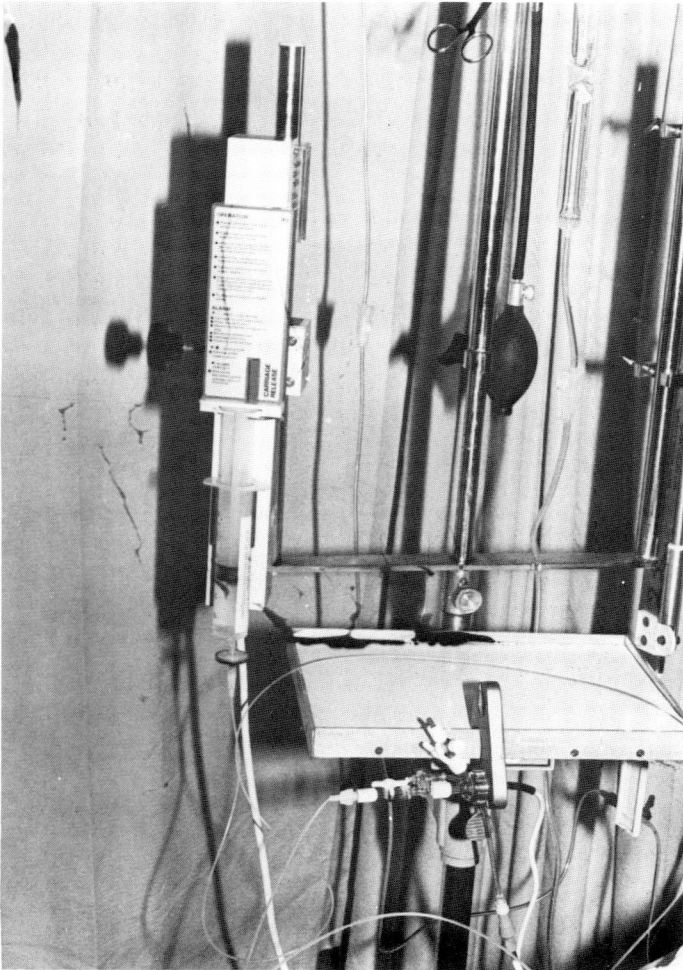

Fig. 5.1 *An infusion pump attached to an unseen patient. This pump is delivering morphine intravenously at a continuous, known rate.*

the required level of analgesia can be readily maintained. It is most frequently used for patients with severe postoperative pain such as that after major abdominal or thoracic surgery.

Drugs used for intravenous infusion

By far the commonest drug used for this purpose is morphine and, although others have been tried, they have as a rule been less successful and reliable.

Inhalation Analgesia

This method of analgesia is only occasionally used in the recovery room but it is of value as a short and rapidly-acting supplement to other forms of analgesia such as intravenous or intramuscular morphine. It is therefore suitable for the provision of additional analgesia when a painful procedure is being carried out, such as chest physiotherapy in patients who have had abdominal or chest surgery.

Nitrous oxide is now the most important and frequently used agent for this purpose and it is supplied in a mixture of 50% nitrous oxide and 50% oxygen in specially prepared cylinders. This preparation is called *Entonox*. It is administered to the patient through a face mask (Fig. 5.2). Fifty per cent of nitrous oxide, when inhaled for several minutes, will produce a good level of analgesia and, although the patient may become drowsy, he will still be able to cooperate with nursing and medical staff and physiotherapist. The Entonox cylinder is fitted with a special type of valve so that the gas mixture is delivered only when the patient takes a breath. This is called a demand valve and is opened by the negative pressure of the patient's inspiration.

If necessary, the anaesthetist may administer 60–70% nitrous oxide with oxygen to provide a greater degree of analgesia. An anaesthetic machine is required to provide these higher concentrations of nitrous oxide. The drowsiness associated with the inhalation of nitrous oxide disappears within a few minutes of stopping inhalation of the gas.

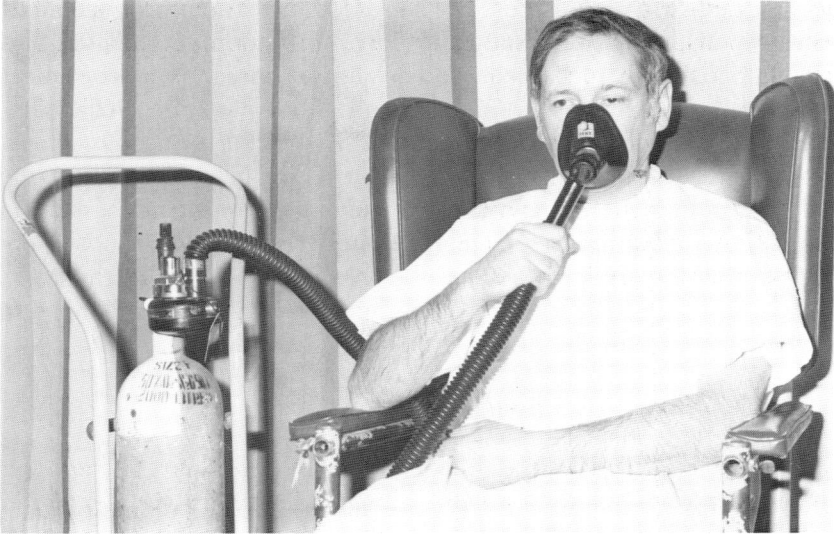

Fig. 5.2 *A patient inhaling Entonox before receiving physiotherapy.*

Nerve Blocks

Nerves or groups of nerves, such as the brachial plexus, may be temporarily blocked by injecting local anaesthetic solutions close to the nerves, thus producing anaesthesia in the area supplied by the nerves. This is a procedure which is frequently carried out for certain forms of surgery, e.g. surgery on the hand under a brachial plexus block. It is rarely used purely as a method of producing postoperative analgesia. It has been shown, however, that patients with brachial plexus blocks experience less pain and require much less analgesic drug postoperatively, hence such a local or regional block is a valuable adjunct to postoperative comfort.

Intercostal nerve blocks can be administered in the recovery room for patients who have had abdominal or thoracic operations. An intercostal nerve is blocked by injecting local anaesthetic solution alongside the nerve as it runs under the rib. The injection is usually made posteriorly at the angle of the rib. Multiple injections are required since several intercostal nerves must be blocked bilaterally to produce analgesia over an area wide enough to cover an operative incision, and the injections have to be repeated at regular intervals as the effect of the local anaesthetic solution wears off. They have the further disadvantage that if the lung is punctured a pneumothorax may occur. Furthermore, the patient has to sit up or lie on his side to allow the block to be administered, and this may be undesirable. Such a method is therefore of very limited value and is only rarely used for postoperative pain. Intercostal blocks may be injected from inside the chest by the surgeon before closure of a thoracotomy. This will help to provide analgesia for the first few hours postoperatively.

Regional Blocks

The most frequently used regional block for postoperative analgesia is the *epidural block*. This involves the injection of a volume of local analgesic solution into the epidural space, which is the space that exists between the two layers of the dura mater surrounding the spinal cord within the bony spinal canal. The spinal nerves pass through this space and can be blocked by local anaesthetic drugs injected into the space. Using full aseptic techniques, a specially designed needle (Tuohy Needle) (Fig. 5.3) is passed between two of the vertebral spines so that its tip enters the epidural space. Certain methods are used to identify entry of the needle into the space. A fine catheter (Fig. 5.3) is passed through the needle (Fig. 5.4) so that several centimetres of the catheter lie in the epidural space and the needle is then removed over the catheter leaving the catheter in place (Fig. 5.5, Fig. 5.6). A bacterial filter is attached to the end of the catheter to minimise the risk of infection (Fig. 5.7). Local anaesthetic solution can now be injected through the catheter and will produce analgesia in the region supplied by the spinal nerves which pass through the area affected by the anaesthetic. The extent of the area affected depends on the volume of anaesthetic solution injected. The solutions used are usually lignocaine 1–2%, or bupivacaine 0.25–0.5%. Bupivacaine has a longer duration of action and one injection may last up to 5 hours, whereas lignocaine will last only 2 to 3 hours; consequently bupivacaine is now becoming more popular.

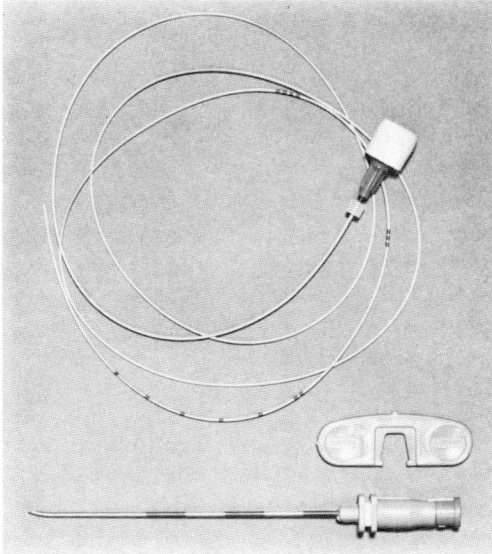

Fig. 5.3 *An 18-gauge Tuohy needle. Note the curvature at the tip of the needle. A detachable 'wing' is adjacent to the hub of the needle. This can be attached to the hub near its junction with the shaft of the needle and can be used to help control the forward movement of the needle through the tissues. An epidural catheter is also shown, above.*

Recently, attention has been given to the injection of certain specially prepared solutions of narcotic analgesic agents, especially morphine, into the epidural space. The results of such studies are at present under evaluation.

The level of the spinal column at which the catheter is inserted is determined by the site of the operation; to provide analgesia for a lower abdominal operation, for example, the catheter would be inserted into the lumbar region, and to provide analgesia for a thoracotomy at the 5th and 6th intercostal space the catheter would be inserted into the lower thoracic region.

The catheter is best inserted before the operation is started so that the epidural block can be used to provide analgesia during the operation as well as postoperatively. It can be left in place for up to 3 days, by which time the worst of the pain will be over.

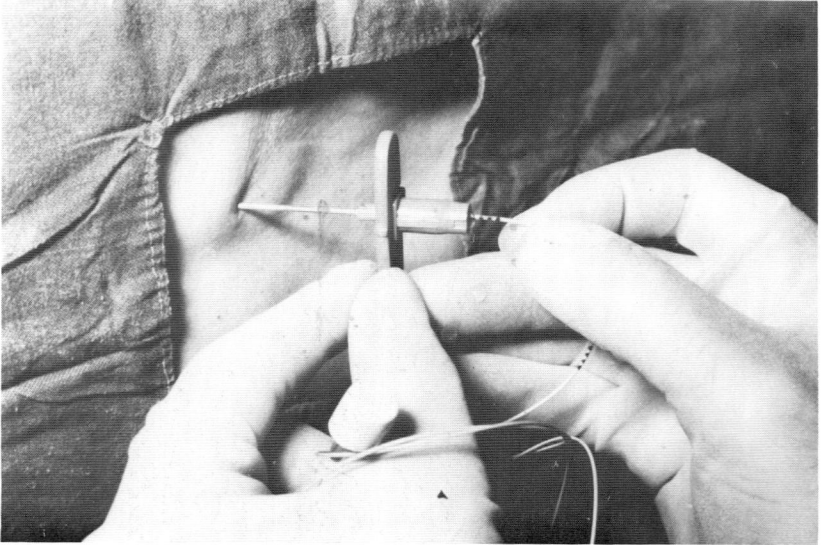

Fig. 5.4 *The epidural catheter being passed through the needle into the epidural space.*

There are certain disadvantages and dangers of epidural analgesia. As well as producing blockade of the nerve fibres which carry pain impulses, there may be blockade of the motor fibres and thus the patient will experience a degree of paralysis of the legs while the epidural is effective. In addition, the sympathetic nerve fibres which control the calibre of blood vessels will be blocked and therefore there will be widespread vasodilatation below the level of the block. This will produce reduction of the blood pressure and it is important that a freely-running intravenous drip should be in place so that intravenous fluids may be given rapidly to reverse hypotension if necessary. It follows from this that an epidural block should not be induced in a patient who may be suffering from a low blood volume due to haemorrhage or dehydration. It also follows that any blood loss occurring while an epidural is effective should be fully replaced since the patient's sympathetic system will not be able to compensate for the blood loss by causing vasoconstriction in the usual way. One of the

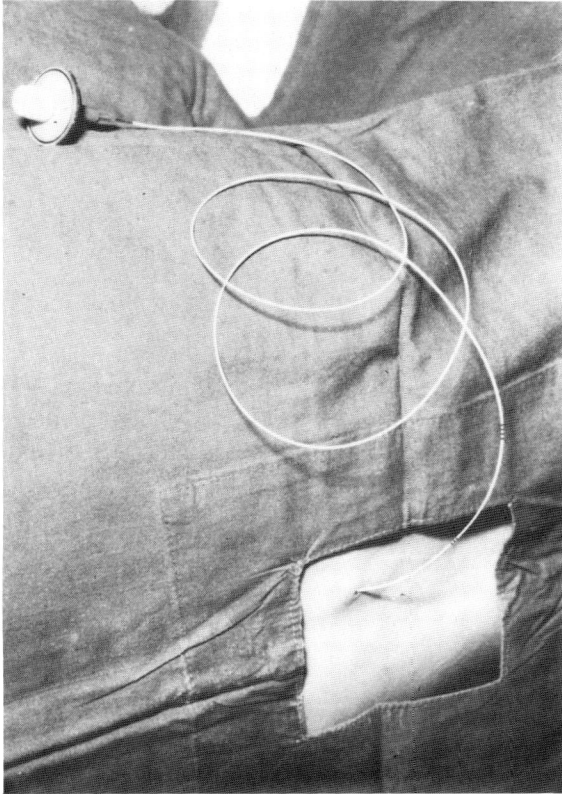

Fig. 5.5 *The epidural catheter in place with the Tuohy needle having been removed. To do this, the Luer connector is removed from the end of the catheter and the Tuohy needle slid along the catheter and off the end. The Luer connector is then replaced and a bacterial filter attached as shown.*

advantages claimed for epidural narcotics is that they do not cause blockade of the sympathetic nerves and hence are much less likely to produce hypotension than the local anaesthetic drugs.

The major advantage of epidural analgesia is that total pain relief can be achieved and the patient does not require supplementary analgesia for nursing procedures and physiotherapy. He is alert and able to cooperate well.

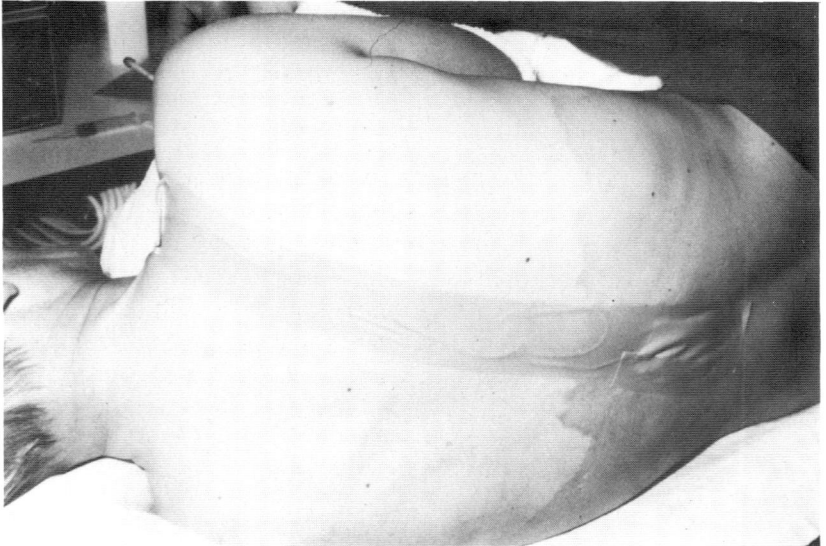

Fig. 5.6 *The epidural catheter is led up to the patient's shoulder and taped to his back to minimise the risk of accidental removal.*

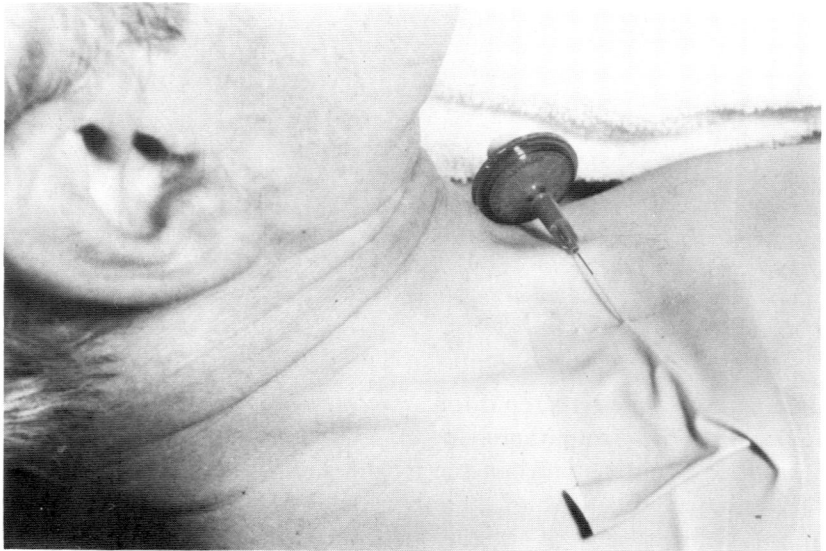

Fig. 5.7 *The end of the epidural catheter with bacterial filter attached is secured at the patient's shoulder thus giving easy access for top-up doses of local anaesthetic.*

'Top-up' doses of analgesic solution should, where possible, be given before the previous dose wears off. This does not result in a wider spread of analgesia but simply reinforces the analgesia already present.

At the present time, the only nurses permitted to give top-up doses are State Certified Midwives who are experienced in supervising patients with epidural analgesia in labour. Thus, in the general recovery room, top-up doses will be given by medical staff, usually an anaesthetist. Epidural analgesia is well established as a means of providing good analgesia for pregnant women in labour and for Caesarean section. It has the major advantage that it will produce good analgesia for the mother without the use of narcotic drugs which may produce respiratory depression in the newly-born baby.

Oral Analgesics

Patients who have had minor surgery under local or regional anaesthesia are often able to take drugs orally soon after the operation and therefore analgesic agents may be administered in this way as the local anaesthetic begins to wear off. The type of drug required may vary from mild analgesia such as soluble aspirin (in solution; 600–900 mg for an adult) to much more powerful agents such as pethidine (50–100 mg for an adult) or buprenorphine which may be given sublingually (0.3–0.6 mg for an adult). Buprenorphine is not recommended for children.

Some patients who have had minor surgery of short duration under general anaesthesia may also be suitable for the administration of oral analgesic agents.

Drugs for oral consumption by adults are usually prepared in standard-size tablets and therefore administration of such drugs on a patient–weight basis is difficult. This difficulty has, to some extent, been overcome for children by the use of solutions or suspensions of analgesic drugs such as paracetamol elixir.

After major surgery, oral analgesic drugs may be used when the period of immediate severe postoperative pain is over, provided the patient is permitted oral intake.

The Nurse's Duties in Relation to Pain Relief

Pain is often accompanied by anxiety, and one of the important duties of the nurse is to reassure the patient. An attempt must be made by the nurse to assess how much pain the patient is experiencing and thus to assess when further doses of analgesic are required. The assessment of pain is extremely difficult since patients react very differently to it.

Nurses will be required to give drugs which are prescribed for oral or intramuscular administration; when drugs are given intravenously a doctor will have to administer them. If an intravenous infusion of analgesic drug is in progress, the nurse will be required to supervise the infusion pump to see that the settings for the infusion rate are correct, that the pump is functioning properly, and that the drug is being delivered to the patient without leakage from the infusion line.

When an epidural is being used, close observation of blood pressure and pulse are required for the reasons stated on p. 64.

If given in excess, narcotic analgesic agents given intramuscularly and intravenously, as well as drugs given by the epidural route, can cause *respiratory depression* and changes in respiratory pattern (*see* Chapter 8). The nurse must therefore report to a member of the medical staff any undue slowing in respiratory rate or change in respiratory pattern.

CHAPTER 6

Oxygen Therapy

The Need for Oxygen Postoperatively

Within the normal, healthy lung there is a fairly constant relationship between the amount of air which is breathed in and the amount of blood which is pumped through the lungs by the right ventricle. This relationship is known as the *ventilation/perfusion ratio* $(\dot{V}/Q)$. It is normally about 4/5. This means that for every 4 l of air which enter the alveoli there are 5 l of blood passing through the lung capillaries to take up oxygen and give up carbon dioxide. This relationship results in the patient having normal arterial oxygen and carbon dioxide tensions in his blood.

When a pathological condition occurs within the lung there is almost always an upset in the $\dot{V}/Q$ ratio. For example, if a patient develops lobar pneumonia, the alveoli in the affected part of the lung will be partially or completely filled with infected secretions, pus and blood. Air cannot therefore enter these alveoli and so the pneumonic area is poorly ventilated. On the other hand, it is still perfused by blood and so obviously there is a considerable upset in the $\dot{V}/Q$ ratio for that part of the lung. The effect of failure to ventilate the pneumonic area is that blood flowing through the area takes up no oxygen and gives up little of its carbon dioxide. This has the effect of reducing the P_{O_2} and increasing the P_{CO_2} in the blood leaving the lungs. This is called an *intrapulmonary shunt* since the effect is as though the blood going through the diseased area had been shunted past the lungs directly from the right to the left side of the heart. The elevation of the P_{CO_2} in the arterial blood causes the respiratory centre to be stimulated to increase the total lung ventilation, hence the patient with pneumonia breathes rapidly. The increase in ventilation allows

healthy alveoli to be ventilated more than usual and so the excess carbon dioxide can be removed through them. However, virtually all of
the oxygen in the blood is attached to haemoglobin and, once the
haemoglobin is fully saturated, the blood cannot take up more oxygen.
In this case, since the haemoglobin in blood coming from a healthy
area of lung will already be fully saturated with oxygen, increasing
the ventilation and hence the alveolar Po_2 will not cause the blood
to take up significantly more oxygen. If, on the other hand, as is likely,
there are areas of lung which are ventilated less well than normally,
by increasing the Po_2 in these alveoli, the amount of oxygen transferred to the blood can be increased. The most convenient way of
increasing alveolar Po_2 is to administer oxygen to the patient. This
will increase the saturation of haemoglobin in blood leaving poorly-
ventilated areas of lung and will increase the Po_2 in blood leaving well-
ventilated areas. Hence there will be an overall increase in the amount
of oxygen carried by the haemoglobin.

It is now well recognised that patients who have undergone general
anaesthesia almost invariably have upsets in their $\dot{V}/Q$ relationship
and that the extent of the upset varies with the nature and duration
of the anaesthesia. For example, a brief anaesthetic during which the
patient breathes spontaneously will produce only a minor upset in $\dot{V}/Q$
ratio and this will quickly correct itself. A prolonged anaesthetic, on
the other hand, will allow small areas of alveolar collapse to occur and
produce multiple small areas of upset $\dot{V}/Q$ which may cause a considerable reduction of the patient's arterial Po_2 postoperatively. There
will also be areas where ventilation will be inadequate relative to
perfusion.

If these effects are marked, the administration of oxygen will be
beneficial to the patient and it is now a routine matter in many hospitals that patients should receive oxygen after major or prolonged surgery. Since the $\dot{V}/Q$ upsets under consideration may take a number
of hours to correct themselves, oxygen will in some cases be required
for up to 12 hours postoperatively. This means that oxygen therapy
may have to be continued in the ward after discharge from the
recovery area. If there is doubt as to whether the oxygen should be
discontinued, then the arterial Po_2 should be checked and this will
give an indication of the adequacy of oxygenation.

How much oxygen?

Those patients who receive oxygen as a routine measure after a major operation are usually given 30–40% of oxygen to breathe. Others may require more, such as those with lung or heart disease, or some may require less, for example those with severe chronic obstructive airways disease and emphysema. These special categories of patients should have their blood gases checked pre-operatively to obtain information on their normal Po_2 and Pco_2. They should also be checked immediately postoperatively to see if oxygen therapy is adequate and ventilation satisfactory.

Methods of Administration of Oxygen

The oxygen mask

The oxygen mask is by far the commonest method of administering oxygen (Fig. 6.1).

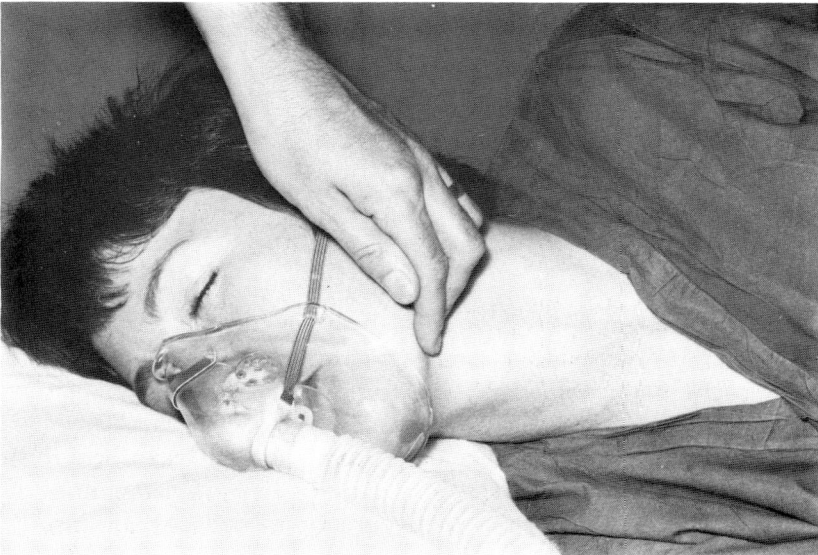

Fig. 6.1 *'Patient' breathing oxygen from a face mask.*
Note that appropriate positioning and airway support are still provided.

Most masks are made of light plastic material so that discomfort for the wearer is minimised. Nevertheless, many patients dislike wearing an oxygen mask and the nurse should ensure that the patient does not remove it.

Modern masks are usually designed so that a small flow of oxygen (say 2–6 l/min) will give a predetermined percentage of oxygen inside the mask. The oxygen entrains air into the mask and is thus diluted to the required level.

Some masks have an adjustable *air entrainment* inlet which allows the oxygen percentage to be varied (Fig. 6.2).

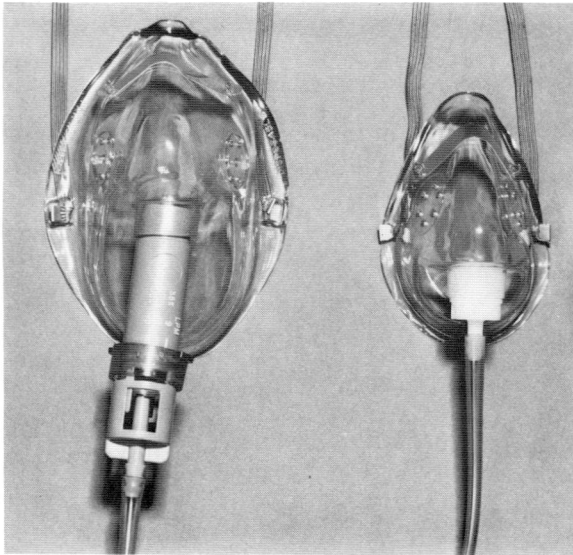

Fig. 6.2 *Oxygen masks, adult and child sizes. The adult mask has an adjustable air entrainment device which allows the inspired oxygen percentage to be adjusted.*

It is important to remember that although a mask can be adjusted to give a predetermined level of oxygen, say 40%, the amount of oxygen entering the patient's respiratory tract may be less than this. This is because the mask provides only a very small reservoir of the air–oxygen mixture and, if the patient's inspiratory air flow is rapid, it will exceed the rate at which oxygen and air are flowing into the mask.

There will therefore be a further dilution of the oxygen by air drawn in from the surrounding atmosphere and the patient may inhale less than the desired amount of oxygen. This can be compensated for by increasing the pre-set oxygen percentage to, say, 50%. The extent of dilution of the oxygen in the mask will also vary according to the closeness of fit of the mask to the patient's face. This obviously varies to a certain extent from patient to patient because of different facial shapes.

Other methods of administering oxygen

Because of surgery to the face, a mask may be unsuitable for some patients. In these circumstances it may be possible to insert a fine catheter through the nose into the pharynx and supply a low flow of oxygen, say two litres per minute, through this. The oxygen is then diluted by the patient's inspired air to give an acceptable level of inspired oxygen. This method has the disadvantage that the inspired percentage of oxygen is unknown.

If the patient has in place or will accept a nasopharyngeal airway, a connector can be attached to the airway and oxygen supplied in known concentration through this. A suitable type of connector is a *'T' piece* (Fig. 6.3). A wide-bore tube carrying the oxygen supply is

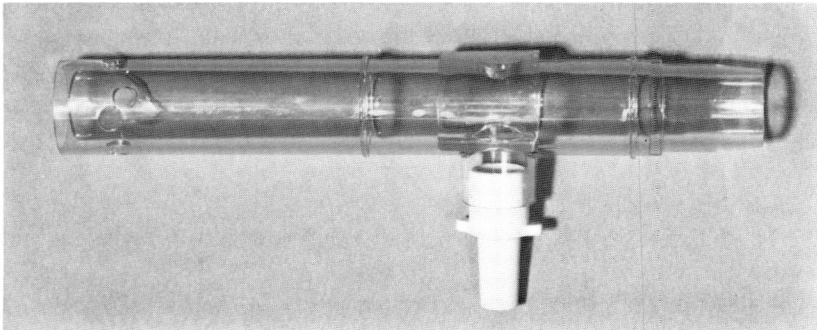

Fig. 6.3 *A 'T' piece attachment. The oxygen supply is connected by wide-bore tubing to the short limb on the right (See Figs 4.8, 4.9, 4.10). The longer limb on the left acts as a small reservoir of oxygen and the vertical limb (with the white connector attached) can be connected to a tracheal tube, a tracheostomy tube, or a nasopharyngeal airway.*

connected to one of the cross-limbs of the 'T'. The other cross-limb has a short piece of wide-bore tubing connected. This forms a reservoir limb. The upright limb of the 'T' is connected to the patient's airway. He can thus breathe freely from a predetermined oxygen supply which is passing through the cross-limb of the 'T'.

A similar 'T' piece arrangement is suitable for patients who have a tracheal tube in place.

Small infants who require oxygen will need to be nursed in an incubator in which the oxygen percentage can be regulated.

Patients who need artificial ventilation for a period after surgery will have the appropriate amount of oxygen administered by adjustment of the percentage of oxygen delivered by the ventilator.

Humidification of oxygen

Oxygen from a cylinder or pipeline contains no water vapour. This is in contrast to normal atmospheric air which always has a certain amount of moisture in it, the amount depending on the relative humidity of the day. The relative humidity is in turn dependent largely on climatic conditions. A recovery room may have air-conditioning which will regulate the temperature and humidity in the room and keep it fairly constant.

During normal breathing, atmospheric air picks up moisture from the mucous membranes of the nose, mouth and other parts of the upper respiratory tract as it is breathed in. The amount of moisture thus added to the air is such that, by the time the air reaches the alveoli, it is almost completely saturated with water vapour. Furthermore, it will be warmed to body temperature.

If a high percentage of oxygen is required, it will be seen that, because of its dryness, a fairly large amount of moisture will be required to saturate it with water vapour. If it is not humidified before it reaches the patient then this moisture will come from the patient's upper respiratory tract. Thus, there will be a drying effect on the mucous membranes of the respiratory tract. This is uncomfortable for the patient and also—because the mucous membranes of the trachea and larger bronchi will become dry—the *cilia*, which normally propel the mucus upwards towards the mouth, cease to work. Secretions are therefore not removed from the respiratory tract and may become a site of infection.

Low percentages of oxygen (up to 40%) will not require humidi-fication since this represents only an increase of 20% of dry oxygen to the inspired air. Higher percentages than this should be humidified. Numerous devices are available for humidifying oxygen. The oxygen passes through the humidifier and either water vapour or a fine mist of water droplets is added to the oxygen stream and is thus carried to the patient.

CHAPTER 7

Fluid Balance and Blood Replacement

Fluid Balance

Patients who are having elective surgery carried out during the morning part of the operating session have, as a rule, had no food or fluid intake since the previous evening. If the operation commences at about 11 a.m. then more than 12 hours will have passed since the last fluid intake. This may be several hours longer if the patient is a young child since he will have gone to sleep earlier than an adult. Thus, many patients who come for elective surgery are already in a certain amount of *fluid deficit.*

If the kidneys are functioning normally, urine output will be decreased, body fluids will be conserved and the deficit will be minimised.

When the surgery is of a minor nature, where the patient can begin to drink within a few hours, the fluid deficit will rapidly be made up and will be of little importance.

If, on the other hand, the surgery is of such a nature as to require that the patient has no oral intake for perhaps several days postoperatively (many operations on the gastrointestinal tract are in this category), then steps should be taken to prevent any serious fluid deficit from occurring. This will involve the administration of fluids by the intravenous route, which will usually have been commenced by the anaesthetist in the operating theatre. In this way, any existing fluid deficit can be made up and subsequent fluid loss can be replaced as it occurs until the patient can take fluids by mouth.

Estimation of Fluid Requirement

In health, fluid output always balances fluid intake. Obviously, under normal living conditions, the amount of fluid drunk or included in food varies greatly from day to day for any individual. It is therefore obvious that, to maintain the balance of intake and output, the output of fluid must vary. The variation in output is brought about by the kidneys which are able to regulate the amount of fluid excreted as urine so that the balance is maintained.

Other fluid losses occur which are not under the control of body systems. Fluid is lost from the respiratory tract. This is the fluid which is taken up to humidify the inspired air. It will obviously vary a certain amount depending on the humidity of the inspired air but is usually in the region of 0.5 1/24 hours.

Fluid is also lost as *insensible perspiration,* i.e. fluid evaporation from the skin which the individual is unaware of. This is also in the region of 0.5 1/24 hours. Sensible perspiration also occurs and is a very variable quantity. A labourer doing hard manual work on a warm summer day may lose several litres of fluid as perspiration and this will have to be made up by increased fluid intake. An office worker in an air-conditioned office, on the other hand, may lose little in the way of sensible perspiration.

A patient in hospital is in a fairly well controlled environment as far as temperature and humidity are concerned and the fluid requirement for an average adult will be about 3 1/24 hours. This will make up for obligatory losses from skin and respiratory tract and also give an adequate urine output.

The *urine output* is an important indicator of the adequacy of fluid replacement and it should be possible to maintain a minimum urine output of at least 30 ml/hour. This is easy to measure in patients who have a urinary catheter in place but in other patients the hourly output has to be estimated from the quantity of urine voided at intervals by the patient.

A *fluid balance chart,* showing all fluid intake and measurable fluid loss, should be kept from the morning of operation. Patients who have had abnormal fluid losses will already be on a fluid balance chart prior to the day of operation.

Measurable fluid losses

Urine will be the main fluid lost. Its volume must be measured. If a catheter is in place, measurement of urine drainage into a suitable graduated container is easy. If there is any reason to be concerned about the patient's renal function, either because of pre-existing kidney disease or as a result of the surgery, the patient should be catheterised and the volume of urine produced each hour should be recorded. If the patient's fluid input has been adequate before, during and after surgery, a urine output of at least 30 ml/hour should be maintained. Volumes below this will alert the nurse to the possibility of the onset of an acute renal problem which, if confirmed by other tests, will require special management. It must be said, however, that the commonest cause of low urine volume postoperatively is inadequate fluid intake. If, for example, a patient has nothing to drink from 9 p.m. or 10 p.m. on the evening before his operation, empties his bladder on the morning of his operation. and then is unable to drink until mid-afternoon, he will produce only a small quantity of highly-concentrated urine postoperatively unless he is given fluid by the intravenous route.

Gastric contents

Some patients will be nauseated and will vomit after anaesthesia and surgery. Usually this is a short-lived phenomenon but the volume of fluid vomited should, where possible, be measured. Many patients having intra-abdominal surgery, especially to the gastrointestinal tract, will come to the recovery area with a nasogastric tube in place. Intra-abdominal surgery is often associated with a period of inactivity of the bowel which may last for several days. During this period, the normal gastric and intestinal secretions collect within the stomach and the intestine and do not pass along the intestinal tract in the normal manner. Similarly, gases which are produced during the normal digestive processes collect within the bowel and cause abdominal distension and discomfort. Patients in this condition (which is called *'paralytic ileus'*) tend to be very uncomfortable and nauseated. A nasogastric tube may help to releive the nausea by allowing gastric fluid to drain continuously into a drainage bag. This gastric fluid should be measured and its volume replaced intravenously.

Intestinal fluids

These may be lost in fairly large quantities if a patient develops diarrhoea in the postoperative period and although the volume may be difficult to measure, especially if the patient is incontinent of faeces, an adequate allowance must be made in the patient's regime of fluid intake.

Certain operations on the intestine will result in the patient having an ileostomy or a colostomy. This means that an end of bowel will be brought out on to the skin surface of the abdomen and sutured in position. This may be temporary or permanent depending on the nature of the patient's illness. Regardless of the causes of the ileostomy, there will be a certain amount of fluid loss from it and this should be collected in a specially designed ileostomy bag and measured.

Loss of fluid into the intestine

As mentioned above, patients who develop paralytic ileus will continue to secrete fluid into the bowel. This also occurs in patients who develop intestinal obstruction. Many patients who develop acute intestinal obstruction will require emergency surgery as a life-saving procedure to relieve the obstruction. Patients who suffer a perforated abdominal viscus (e.g. a perforated duodenal ulcer, or a ruptured viscus resulting from abdominal injury) will also rapidly develop a paralytic ileus after the perforation or injury. All patients in this group will lose fluid into the bowel lumen which is not quickly reabsorbed, and so they will be in *fluid deficit*. The amount of deficit will depend on the duration of the illness, and may be several litres. Thus, the patient requiring emergency surgery may be grossly dehydrated and his circulating blood volume will be low. Attempts should be made to correct the deficit as far as possible before surgery but this may not always be possible and, of course, the paralytic ileus will persist after surgery and intravenous fluids will be required to correct the fluid deficit. Fluid in the bowel cannot be measured, and so the adequacy of its replacement must be estimated by other methods. These are described on pp. 82–83.

Fluid loss from surgical drains

Frequently, especially after certain types of abdominal operation, and always after intrathoracic operations, it can be anticipated that there will be blood or other fluids coming from the site of operation, and so the surgeon will insert a drain leading from the operation site out through the skin surface to allow the fluid to drain out. This drain may come out either through the wound or, more usually, through a seperate small incision. Such a drain may be a tube to which suction can be attached to help remove fluid, or it may be simply a piece of corrugated plastic or rubber if the operation is superficial, such as when a breast lump has been removed. Drains from the chest cavity are always led to a one-way valvular system such as a *water seal drain* which allows fluid (and air) to drain out of the chest but does not allow air to be sucked into the chest when the patient breathes in.

Types of fluid removed through drains

Where possible the volume of any fluid drained should be measured and charted, along with a note as to its nature, e.g. blood, bile, etc. The fluid most commonly drained is blood. All operations are associated with a certain amount of blood loss but it can be anticipated in some cases that blood will continue to be lost after the operation is over. Such operations include most intrathoracic procedures, operations on the prostate gland, certain major orthopaedic operations, major plastic operations around the face and neck, breast operations and certain intra-abdominal operations, especially those involving the liver. Where the operation has been necessary because of trauma, especially where there are multiple injuries with widespread tissue damage, the postoperative blood loss may be considerable and may occur from more than one site.

Bile may be drained after certain operations involving the liver and biliary tract.

Drains are often inserted where there is soiling of the peritoneal cavity by intestinal contents, for example after an operation to repair a perforated duodenal ulcer. The volume of fluid drained may vary from a few millilitres in all to several hundred millilitres per day, depending on the nature and duration of contamination of the peritoneum and whether or not infection has occurred.

Fluid loss may occur through the operation wound, in which case it will be absorbed in the dressing. Again, blood is the fluid most commonly lost in this way and its volume will be impossible to measure.

Excessive blood loss appearing through drains or on dressings means that the patient is continuing to bleed excessively or has started to bleed since the end of the operation. It may be necessary in such circumstances to return the patient to the operating theatre and re-open the wound to achieve control of the bleeding surgically.

Estimation of Fluid Requirements

The patient's fluid intake must be adjusted to take account of all fluid losses. These include :

1. *Insensible losses*
   - through the respiratory tract (500 ml/day);
   - through the skin (500 ml/day);
2. *Other*
   - through the skin as perspiration (a variable amount);
   - urine (a variable amount but easily measured);
   - additional losses from gastrointestinal tract, through drainage and on to dressings, etc. (some can be measured, some must be estimated).

Where the surgery is minor and no excess fluid loss expected, the patient will be able to drink soon after surgery and will rapidly adjust his own fluid intake to his requirements.

After major surgery (especially to the bowel), when the patient may be unable to take fluids orally for several days, his fluid requirements must be given intravenously by drip. An adult with well-functioning kidneys may safely be given 3 l/24 hours. This will make up for insensible losses and provide a good volume of urine (more than 30 ml/hour). This 3 l volume is usually made up of standard solutions of commercially prepared, sterile solutions which are available in litre and half-litre quantities. A regime of 2 l of 5% dextrose and 1 l of 0.9% sodium chloride (normal saline) is commonly used initially. The fluid is infused intravenously at a rate of 1 1/8 hours, alternating the dextrose and saline solutions. The regime of fluids to be infused must be prescribed by a member of the medical staff.

Patients who have abnormal fluid losses (i.e. from the gastro-intestinal tract or by drains) will need to have these abnormal losses made up by infusion of additional volumes of fluid; this means that a doctor will have to alter the prescription for intravenous fluids.

Although much of the volume of fluid lost will be measurable, normally some of it is not and, if the amount which cannot be measured is large, there is a danger of the patient developing a deficiency of fluid since the volume of fluid loss usually tends to be underestimated. In this situation, in addition to measuring fluid losses as far as possible and replacing these, other means are used to estimate the adequacy of fluid replacement.

Indications of Fluid Deficiency

Urine volume

When fluid intake is inadequate to meet fluid losses, the body responds by conserving fluid. This is done by the kidneys, which will excrete a low volume of urine. Since the usual quantities of products of metabolism (i.e. urea, etc) still have to be excreted, the urine will contain a higher concentration than usual. The first indication of fluid deficit is therefore the passage of a low volume of highly concentrated urine. If the fluid deficit is allowed to persist, and to become severe, there will be a rising pulse rate and a fall in central venous pressure and the patient will begin to look unwell. This appearance is due to tissue *dehydration*. If this is allowed to continue the eyes look sunken and the skin is dry and loses its normal elastic properties. Finally, as dehydration progresses, biochemical changes occur in the blood, with rising blood urea and abnormalities in electrolyte levels. If post-operative care is good, no patient should ever approach this state as a result of dehydration.

Fluid Replacement: Routes of Intake

Oral

The majority of patients will be able to drink a few hours after surgery and retain the fluid without vomiting. As a rule, such patients do not need special fluid regimes and can be allowed to drink freely. They will soon make up any existing fluid deficit resulting from having no fluid intake since the night before.

Nasogastric tube

Certain operations render patients temporarily unable to swallow, for example major operations within the mouth and in the neck region. If the patient's bowel is working normally (as it should be after such operations), a plastic tube can be passed through the nose, down the oesophagus and into the stomach (a nasogastric tube Fig. 4.10). The patient's fluids and nutrition can then be administered through the tube and will pass directly into the stomach. Solid food can be taken but needs to be liquidised so that it can pass down the tube. Alternatively, commercially prepared nutritive mixtures are available for nasogastric feeding.

The nasogastric method makes use of the normal bowel for absorbing fluids and nutrition and is therefore preferable to intravenous administration of fluids.

Intravenous route

When a patient is unable to have fluids orally, or by nasogastric tube, the intravenous route must be used. This requires the setting up of an intravenous drip (or infusion). If it is anticipated that the drip will be required for only a day or two, a peripheral vein is used, usually in the arm or hand. This is set up by a doctor. The site chosen for the drip is usually where a large vein is easily visible superficially. The forearm is preferable to the elbow or the hand because the forearm does not bend and therefore does not require to be splinted, and, if well secured by sticky tape, the drip cannula will not be easily dislodged. This is more comfortable for the patient and allows limited use of the hand.

If the arm is hairy, the area around the drip site should be shaved and then thoroughly cleaned using an antiseptic solution. The doctor setting up the drip should scrub his hands and wear sterile gloves.

A small volume of local anaesthetic solution is infiltrated into the skin at the puncture site (0.5 ml of 0.5% lignocaine is suitable) and the vein is punctured using a 16- or 18-gauge cannula (in an adult), preferably of the Teflon type. Teflon is preferred because it slides easily through skin and is non-irritant to tissues. When the cannula is in position, the metal needle is withdrawn from it and the giving set, previously primed with the fluid to be infused, is connected to the hub of the cannula. The fluid is allowed to run into the vein to check the patency of the cannula and also to check that the fluid is not leaking out of the vein into the surrounding tissue. A swelling will rapidly occur around the vein if this should happen. If the drip runs satisfactorily, the cannula and lower end of the giving set are fixed securely to the patient's arm with sticky tape. If it has been necessary to use a vein overlying a joint (elbow or wrist), the arm will need to be splinted with the appropriate joint held straight so that the cannula will not be distorted or dislodged. The drip rate should be adjusted so that the prescribed amount of fluid is infused over the appropriate time.

Giving sets have sites incorporated for the injection of drugs and this is often used to avoid further injections and thus discomfort for the patient when drugs have to be given intravenously. Except in special circumstances, drugs may only be given intravenously by doctors.

Long-term Intravenous Infusions: Central Venous Catheterisation

Where it is anticipated that intravenous therapy will be required for more than a few days, it is common practice to insert a catheter into the superior vena cava (SVC). This is done by passing the catheter through a cannula which is inserted into one of the large deep tributary veins of the superior vena cava—usually the internal jugular vein (*see* Fig. 3.4) or subclavian vein. Sometimes the external jugular vein or the antecubital vein at the elbow are used, but it is more difficult to pass a catheter through these into the SVC.

Attempted puncture of the internal jugular vein or subclavian vein carries much greater risks for the patient than a peripheral vein puncture and should be done by a doctor experienced in the technique. Full aseptic technique is necessary since the risk of producing blood-borne infection is greater with a centrally-placed catheter. A chest x-ray must be taken to confirm that the central venous catheter is in the correct position (*see* Fig. 3.4).

Fluids used

Initially the patient will usually receive one of the solutions of 'clear fluid' (dextrose, normal saline or Hartmann's solution). Hartmann's is a solution containing several solutes so that its constitution is more akin than saline to the electrolyte content of human blood. For small infants, special dilute solutions of saline are used. The volumes used are discussed on pp. 82–83.

If clear fluid infusion is used for more than 24 hours then it may be necessary to add other electrolytes to the solution, such as potassium chloride. This requirement is determined on the basis of blood electrolyte values, which should be checked daily for patients having an intravenous fluid regime

If the patient is unable to take nutrition orally or by nasogastric tube for more than 2 or 3 days postoperatively, it may be necessary to commence *intravenous feeding* in order to supply sufficient calories for energy and nitrogen for tissue repair. These are supplied in the form of special commercially-prepared sterile solutions of highly concentrated dextrose (up to 50%) and amino acids. Fat emulsions are also available for intravenous use and are an important source of calories. A regime of nutrition is made up for each patient each day and appropriate electrolyte, vitamin and mineral supplements should be included.

Since most of the intravenous nutritional preparations are highly irritant to the smaller peripheral veins and cause them to thrombose, intravenous nutrition is given through a central venous catheter into the superior vena cava. In the superior vena cava, the solution is rapidly diluted in the large flow of blood and does not cause irritation.

Blood Transfusion

Patients who lose 10% or more of their estimated blood volume should have the blood loss replaced by blood or a blood substitute. Blood of the patient's blood group should be cross-matched beforehand for all patients having major surgery performed or for any procedure where it is anticipated that significant blood loss may occur. The volume of blood prepared should be related to the anticipated loss. Preparation of blood for transfusion requires a specimen of the patient's blood to be sent to the blood transfusion laboratory in the hospital, preferably at least 24 hours before surgery. In the laboratory, the patient's blood group is determined from the specimen and the required number of units of blood of the same group are matched with the patient's blood by using special methods. The correct matching of blood units will help to prevent the patient receiving an incompatible blood transfusion which can have serious and even fatal consequences. Each unit is labelled with the blood group of the donor and, when matched with the blood of a patient, an additional label is attached with the patient's name, address and hospital number.

Administration of blood

When blood is required, it will usually be obvious in the operating theatre and the transfusion will have been commenced there by the anaesthetist. Instructions will be given as to how much more blood the patient should receive postoperatively. Before commencing transfusion of a unit of blood, the labels on the blood unit must be checked against the patient's name, address, hospital number and blood group. This check should be done by two persons at the patient's bedside. *If there is the slightest doubt about a blood unit being the correct one for any patient, it must not be used.*

Warming of blood

In order to preserve blood, it is stored in a refrigerator at 4°C until it is required for transfusion. If a large volume is transfused therefore, it will have a significant cooling effect on the patient and so, if more than two units are required, the blood should be warmed by passing it through a specially designed *blood warmer* (Fig. 7.1). When it reaches the patient it is then almost at 37°C and the cooling effect is minimal.

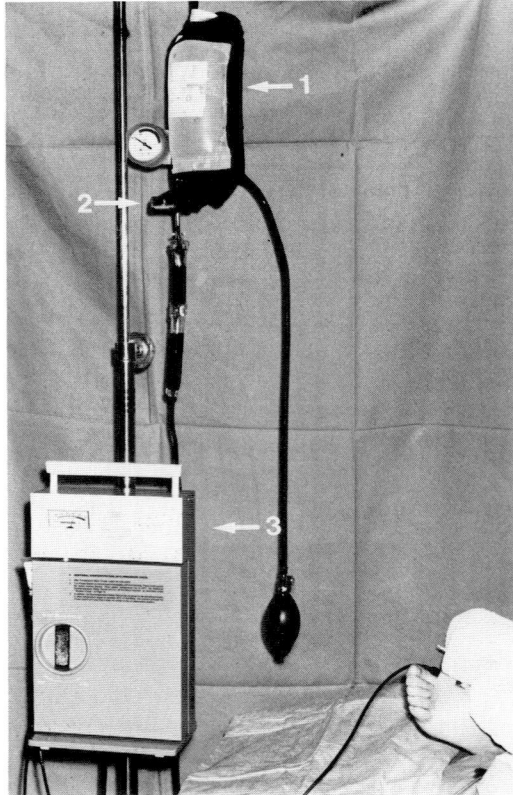

Fig. 7.1 *This shows a blood transfusion in progress. In this case, the cannula has been placed in a vein in the patient's foot because both arms had been involved in the operation. The bag of blood is pressurised using a pressure infusor (1) to increase the rate of transfusion. A blood filter (2) and a blood warmer (3) are also in use.*

Filtration of blood

During storage, small aggregates of platelets and cellular debris accumulate in blood. If a large volume transfusion is given, these aggregates arrive in the lungs where they are retained and can cause lung damage. To minimise this, the blood should be filtered to remove such debris. All giving sets for blood contain a filter, but this has pores which are too large to effectively filter out the micro-aggregates which are under consideration. Filters are available which will filter out the micro-aggregates and these should be used for all blood transfusions. The filter has a nozzle which is inserted into the blood bag (Fig. 7.1). It is then 'primed', i.e. filled with blood from the bag so as to drive out any air which it may contain, and then the giving set is attached to the outlet of the filter.

Concentrated red cells

Many special products are prepared from human blood by the blood transfusion service, such as plasma, human albumin solutions, immunoglobulins and factor VIII (for treatment of haemophilia). This requires large quantities of plasma to be taken from blood and therefore much of the blood supplied to hospitals is depleted of a certain amount of its plasma. Such units of blood are therefore of value in the treatment of certain blood disorders where the requirement is for red cells and where there has not been acute blood loss. When such units are given in the situation of acute blood loss, it must be remembered that they are volume-depleted and an appropriate volume of clear fluid or plasma will be required to make up the volume of blood lost.

Duties of the Nurse in Relation to Fluid Balance

Fluid losses

The nurse must, where possible, measure all fluids lost by the patient. Where fluids are lost, but are not measurable, the attention of the medical staff should be drawn to these so that, between them, the nurse and the doctor may arrive at an estimate of the amount of the fluid loss.

A chart must be kept showing the amount of all fluids lost (urine, blood loss, surgical drains, nasogastric drainage, vomited fluid, and bowel losses—ileostomy, colostomy, bowel movements). The chart should be updated hourly when fluid loss is severe.

Fluid replacement

When intravenous fluids are required, the fluid regime will be prescribed by the medical staff. The nurse must ensure that this regime is adhered to and that each unit of intravenous fluid is given at an even rate over the prescribed time. The time of commencement and completion of each unit of fluid infused should be charted, as well as the numbers of blood units, plasma and clear fluid units.

Care of an intravenous infusion

All intravenous infusions are set up by doctors. In a patient immediately after operation, the infusion will usually have been set up in theatre. Most such infusions will be 'peripheral' drips (i.e. into an arm vein).

The nurse must inspect the drip site regularly to ascertain that there is no leakage of fluid at the junction of the giving set and the intravenous cannula, and to ascertain that the puncture site is not bleeding. The nurse should also check that there is no swelling around the vein in the area of the puncture site. This would indicate that the drip had 'tissued' or 'infiltrated', i.e. that the fluid from the infusion was leaking out into the tissues around the vein. If this occurs, the infusion should be stopped immediately and the situation reported to a member of the medical staff who will, if necessary, restart the infusion at another site.

Care of a central venous line

Because the tip of a central venous catheter lies in a vein within the chest, it will not infiltrate into surrounding tissues. If a central venous infusion ceases to flow it must be assumed that the catheter has become blocked and it will have to be replaced by a doctor.

It is likely that the catheter will have been sutured in place at the skin and the puncture site covered by a sterile dressing. The puncture site should be inspected daily to see if there is evidence of infection or leakage of fluid.

A central venous line is used not only for infusions but also for measuring central venous pressure (CVP) and it is thus subjected to frequent interruptions in the flow of fluid. When the CVP has been checked, the nurse must remember to restart the infusion; otherwise the catheter may become blocked by blood clot. A central venous line must never be disconnected and left open to the air for even a few seconds. If this happens, the negative pressure which is often generated in the central veins during inspiration will cause air to be drawn through the catheter into the superior vena cava and the heart, forming an *air embolus*. If a large air embolus occurs, it will cause obstruction to the flow of blood through the heart, resulting in acute heart failure and cardiac arrest.

CHAPTER 8

Postoperative Respiratory Failure

Some Definitions

Apnoea means absence of breathing.

Respiratory rate means the number of breaths per minute.

Tidal volume is the volume of air in each breath, e.g. 0.5 l.

Minute volume is the volume of air breathed in each minute and is equal to the product of the tidal volume and the respiratory rate. For example, 0.5 l (tidal volume) × 14 (respiratory rate) = 7 l minute volume.

Dead space is that part of the respiratory tract which does not take part in the exchange of oxygen and carbon dioxide between the inspired air and the blood. It includes the nasal passages, the mouth, pharynx, larynx, trachea and bronchi. It is approximately equal to 2 ml/kg of body weight.

Gas exchange is the process by which oxygen enters the blood from the air in the lungs and carbon dioxide passes out from the blood into the air. It takes place in the alveoli of the lungs through the alveolar–capillary membrane.

Alveolar–capillary membrane is the very fine membrane of tissue which separates the alveolar air from the blood in the lung capillaries. It is fine enough for molecules of oxygen and carbon dioxide to pass through freely by a process of simple diffusion.

Postoperative Respiratory Insufficiency

Respiratory insufficiency in the postoperative period is a common occurrence. It gives rise to hypoxia and carbon dioxide retention (respiratory acidosis), and is therefore a life-threatening condition if severe and prolonged. It must be promptly recognised and rapidly and effectively treated.

Recognition of respiratory insufficiency

The most extreme form of respiratory insufficiency is total absence of breathing (apnoea) and this requires the immediate commencement of *artificial respiration*. Apnoea is however usually preceded by a period when breathing is present but inadequate. The patient may be cyanosed and this should immediately alert the nurse to a respiratory problem. If the patient is breathing oxygen however, he may not be cyanosed and yet his breathing may not be adequate to ensure satisfactory clearance of carbon dioxide; that is to say his minute volume is inadequate. This may be because the rate of respiration is too slow or the tidal volume is too small, or both. It is important therefore that attention be paid to the respiratory rate, which should be charted. A rate of less than 10 breaths/min should be brought to the attention of the medical staff.

Patients who are in pain, especially after abdominal or thoracic surgery, will tend to breathe rapidly with a small tidal volume. This is because it is more painful to take deeper breaths. Shallow rapid breaths are much less efficient in terms of gas exchange than deeper breaths at a normal rate. This is because of the dead space. It must be remembered that the air which reaches the alveoli at each breath is the tidal volume minus the air which ventilates the dead space. Thus, if a patient breathes 30 times per minute with a tidal volume of 200 ml then the minute volume is 200×30 ml/min $= 6$ l/min. If however the dead space ventilation is 100 ml then the volume of air reaching the alveoli to take part in gas exchange is $(200-100) \times 30$ ml/min $= 3$ l/min. If the tidal volume is doubled (400 ml) and the respiratory rate halved (15 breaths/min), the total minute volume is still 6 l/min (400×15 ml/min). The dead space ventilation is (100×15) ml/min, i.e. 1.5 l/min, and therefore the alveolar ventilation is 4.5 l/min. Thus, for the same minute volume the slower, deeper respiratory pattern gives a greater alveolar ventilation and is therefore more efficient in delivering oxygen to and removing carbon dioxide from the alveoli.

Causes of respiratory insufficiency

Obstruction

The commonest cause of respiratory inadequacy in the postoperative period is respiratory obstruction. This is usually only partial and normally easily corrected by appropriate positioning of the patient and support of the jaw with or without the use of a pharyngeal airway (*see* Chapter 4).

Central respiratory depression

This may occur as a side-effect of drugs given during anaesthesia, or in the immediate postoperative period. The drugs responsible are most likely to be *narcotic* agents given for analgesia. Drugs such as morphine, pethidine, papaveretum and fentanyl are all potent analgesic agents but all have the disadvantage of producing depression of other central nervous functions, particularly conscious level and respiration. Some also depress the cardiovascular centres in the brain and may cause a fall in blood pressure.

If given during anaesthesia therefore, narcotic analgesic agents may cause a delay in recovery of consciousness, respiratory depression and, in some cases, hypotension. Narcotic respiratory depression typically produces a slow respiratory rate, e.g. 5–6/min, but the respirations may be initially of good tidal volume. Later the tidal volume will become smaller. Some patients are especially sensitive to the effects of narcotic drugs. Central respiratory depression may also result from the effects of inhalational agents administered during anaesthesia.

Treatment of central respiratory depression

Respiratory depression due to narcotic analgesia may be treated by providing artificial ventilation for the patient until the effect of the drug has worn off sufficiently to allow the patient to breathe satisfactorily. Depending on the dose of drug administered, this may take several hours. This method has the advantage that the patient will remain analgesic in the immediate postoperative period. It has the disadvantage that the patient must remain intubated and ventilated much longer than would otherwise be necessary and therefore occupies a bed in the recovery area for an unnecessarily long period. Sometimes it is considered advantageous to artificially ventilate certain patients for a number of hours, or perhaps overnight, after certain major operations, for example after certain cardiac, thoracic or major abdominal operations. In such cases, the respiratory depressant effects of narcotics such as morphine are valuable in helping to remove the patient's own respiratory drive and allowing artificial ventilation to be easily maintained.

The other method of treatment of narcotic-induced respiratory depression is the administration of a drug which will reverse the effects of the narcotic. Two drugs are commonly in use for this purpose. These are *naloxone* and *levallorphan*. Naloxone is prepared by the manufacturers in an ampoule of 0.4 mg for intravenous or intramuscular use and may be given intravenously in doses up to 1.2 mg (i.e. 3 ampoules). The narcotic antagonist effects of naloxone are so specific that, if respiratory depression is not reversed at this dose level, it is highly unlikely that the respiratory depression is due to a narcotic. It can thus be used as a diagnostic test where narcotic overdose is suspected. As well as reversing the respiratory depression of narcotics, naloxone also reverses the analgesic and sedative effects. This is obviously a disadvantage in the postoperative period and the manufacturers recommend that it should be administered in small increments of 0.1–0.2 mg in the hope that analgesia will remain while respiratory depression is reversed. Levallorphan is a less potent *narcotic antagonist* than naloxone but is preferred by some doctors because, compared with naloxone, its anti-analgesic effect is less pronounced relative to its anti-respiratory depressant effect.

Respiratory depression with inhalational anaesthetic agents is much less common than that due to narcotics, but its effects are not reversed by narcotic antagonists. Therefore treatment of this form of respiratory depression requires artificial ventilation until the drug is sufficiently removed from the body through the lungs to allow return of adequate respiration.

Respiratory insufficiency due to muscle relaxant drugs

Muscle relaxant drugs are used during anaesthesia for three purposes.

Firstly, to abolish the muscle tone and function of muscles of the thoracic and abdominal areas, thus allowing good access to these areas for the surgeon without undue pulling with retractors.

Secondly, it may be deemed beneficial by the anaesthetist that the patient should be artificially ventilated during surgery because it is felt that his breathing may be inadequate under anaesthesia. Patients suffering from certain respiratory or cardiac diseases or gross obesity may come into this category. Patients having intrathoracic surgery are always ventilated by the anaesthetist since the lung on the side of the thoracotomy collapses when the thorax is opened by the surgeon and it is important to ensure good ventilation of the other lung if severe hypoxia is to be avoided. Patients having intracranial operations are also ventilated artificially. By doing so, the anaesthetist can help to control the pressure within the cranial cavity. This is because the level of carbon dioxide tension in the blood profoundly affects the amount of blood which flows through the brain; a raised carbon dioxide tension increasing the blood flow and thus the intracranial contents and pressure, and a lowered carbon dioxide tension having the opposite effect. During surgery, the task of the neurosurgeon is made easier if the bulk and pressure of the cranial contents are reduced and so it is important that carbon dioxide tension should not be allowed to rise above normal and indeed a slight reduction is often aimed for. This is achieved by using artificial ventilation to over-ventilate the lungs to a slight extent.

The third reason for using a muscle relaxant drug is to allow the anaesthetist to insert an endotracheal tube into the trachea. This is always done when a patient is to be ventilated artificially during surgery but it may also be done when the patient is to be allowed to breathe spontaneously. For example, in operations around the face and neck (especially in the mouth and nose) where the use of an

anaesthetic face mask would be inconvenient for the access of the surgeon, or where the patient is to be placed face down on the operating
table, a tracheal tube is inserted to ensure that the airway remains
clear.

If an attempt were to be made to insert a tracheal tube into the
trachea of a lightly anaesthetised patient, it would result in coughing
and laryngeal spasm which will cause respiratory obstruction with all
its attendant problems. To avoid this, the patient must either be
anaesthetised deeply or given a muscle relaxant. Either of these techniques will prevent coughing or laryngeal spasm during intubation.
The administration of a muscle relaxant by intravenous injection is
however a much quicker and simpler method than producing deep
anaesthesia, and it is generally used.

Muscle relaxants are of two types, depolarising and non-
depolarising. The depolarising type, such as suxamethonium, stimulates each muscle fibre to contract before it relaxes and becomes
paralysed. Suxamethonium has a short duration of action (up to 3 or
4 minutes) and is therefore used for those situations where the patient
is to be allowed to breathe spontaneously after intubation. Its effect
wears off spontaneously.

The non-depolarising type of relaxants, such as tubo-curarine
('curare'), pancuronium, alcuronium, gallamine and atracurium have
a longer duration of action (30 to 40 minutes) and are therefore
used when artificial ventilation is to be maintained throughout an
operation. The patient may be intubated under the influence of the
non-depolarising relaxant or he may be given suxamethonium for
intubation followed by the non-depolarising relaxant when the effect
of the suxamethonium has begun to wear off. Non-depolarising
relaxants, because of their long duration of action, need to have their
effects reversed at the end of the operation by the administration
of a drug of the anti-cholinesterase group. The drug usually used is
prostigmine. Occasionally, the dose of prostigmine may be inadequate
to produce full clinical reversal of the relaxant and the patient will
only partially regain his muscle power. Such a patient may be unable
to breathe adequately and, if sent to the recovery room in this state,
will require further treatment. Such treatment may simply consist of
a further dose of prostigmine which may rapidly improve the patient's

muscle power. If however this is not effective, the patient will require respiratory support in the form of artificial ventilation until the relaxant wears off or until further treatment is given. Certain circumstances will serve to prolong the effects of non-depolarising relaxants, for example metabolic acidosis or the administration of certain antibiotics. If respiratory inadequacy occurs postoperatively and is thought to be due to prolonged action of relaxants, the diagnosis can be confirmed by the use of a nerve stimulator. This is a piece of apparatus by which an electrical stimulus is applied to the median nerve at the wrist from electrodes on the skin surface. The pattern of response to the stimulus when a muscle relaxant is acting is different from the normal, non-blocked response pattern.

Inadequate analgesia

Pain which is inadequately relieved will often cause a patient to breathe rapidly with shallow breaths. This is most likely to occur where upper abdominal or thoracic surgery has been carried out because larger breaths are much more painful for the patient. The significance of this type of breathing in terms of gas exchange is explained on p. 94.

When a patient whose respiratory function is normally poor (e.g. a patient with *obstructive airways disease*), is operated upon, the respiratory function is made worse by the postoperative upset in ventilation/perfusion relationships within the lung (*see* Chapter 6) and by the rapid shallow breathing due to inadequate pain relief. The combination of these factors may be sufficient to cause respiratory failure. Good postoperative analgesia will help to remove one of these problems and thus help to avoid respiratory difficulty. Epidural analgesia is often the method of choice in these circumstances.

Chronic respiratory disease

This is a frequent cause of failure to breathe adequately after anaesthesia and surgery. It usually occurs in the patient with severe emphysematous changes in the lungs and chronic obstructive disease of the small airways. Such patients are normally severely limited in their exercise tolerance and many of them have had to give up work because of their respiratory disability. They become breathless on even minor exertion and their breathing is often wheezy in character. Chest expansion is poor and the chest has a typical 'barrel' shape, being increased in its anteroposterior diameter and fixed in a position of inspiration because the emphysematous changes in the lungs do not allow proper expiration to occur. Obviously, such patients are very dependent on diaphragmatic and abdominal movement to allow ventilation of their lungs. After abdominal surgery, such movement will be limited if pain is not well relieved. Furthermore, such patients may be very sensitive to the respiratory depressant effects of narcotic analgesic agents and these must be used cautiously.

Patients with severe chronic obstructive airways disease often have a higher than normal $Paco_2$. Instead of the normal $Paco_2$ of 35–45 mmHg they may run between 50 and 60 mmHg. They also have a low Pao_2—often about 60 mmHg instead of the normal 90–100 mmHg. Obviously these patients have very little capacity for overcoming postoperative respiratory difficulty. The upsets in ventilation/perfusion relationships which are to be expected after surgery and anaesthesia may be enough to push them into respiratory failure.

The severely emphysematous patient has long since ceased to respond to the respiratory stimulus of an elevated $Paco_2$ which would make a person with a healthy respiratory system respond by a marked increase in his minute volume. He is dependent on the stimulus of a low Pao_2 to keep him breathing. If such a patient is therefore given enough oxygen to elevate his Pao_2 significantly above his own normal level, he will cease to breathe adequately. His $Paco_2$ will rise even higher and a severe degree of respiratory acidosis will develop. If untreated, this will eventually cause unconsciousness and death. Therefore these patients, if they require oxygen, must have it administered in a very carefully controlled way and in a percentage which will provide a Pao_2 at or about the patient's normal level.

Oxygen masks are available which can be adjusted to give percentages just above that of air, for example 24% or 28%. Such a small increase above the normal atmospheric oxygen concentration of 21% may be all that the patient will tolerate.

Late Causes of Respiratory Failure

Respiratory difficulties may occur several days after an operation. The most likely causes for these are:

1. Postoperative *pneumonia*;
2. Postoperative *pulmonary atalectesis*;
3. *Pulmonary thrombo-embolism*:

Postoperative pneumonia

This tends to occur most often in patients who have undergone abdominal or thoracic operations. It occurs because the patient fails to adequately cough up his secretions and these then form a site of infection in the lung which may develop into pneumonia. The reasons for failure to breathe adequately are discussed earlier in this chapter. Pneumonia gives rise to pyrexia, rapid breathing and, if severe, cyanosis. There may be bloodstained sputum. The arterial oxygen tension will be low. The onset of these signs and symptoms is usually gradual. An x-ray usually confirms the diagnosis. Treatment is with antibiotics and physiotherapy. Oxygen is often also required.

Postoperative pulmonary atalectesis

This occurs when one area of lung collapses because it is not well ventilated by the patient's respirations. It usually arises because the small bronchus leading to the area of collapse becomes blocked by a plug of mucus which the patient cannot cough up. The collapsed area will often become infected and the signs and symptoms are thus the same as those of a pneumonia and the treatment is similar. Often, in the early stages, a bronchoscopy may help to remove the plug of mucus and allow the collapsed area to re-expand.

Pulmonary thrombo-embolism

This is a common cause of sudden postoperative respiratory difficulty and may occur up to 12 days after operation. It occurs when a clot of blood travels from one of the deep veins in the pelvis or legs, passes through the right side of the heart and impacts in a branch of the pulmonary artery in the lungs.

If the clot is large, sudden death may occur because the main pulmonary artery is obstructed and heart failure rapidly occurs. If the clot is smaller and reaches a branch of the pulmonary artery, the patient will suddenly become breathless and will often complain of sudden onset of acute chest pain. He will often cough up blood. His blood gases will show a reduced arterial oxygen tension (Pao_2). There will also often be evidence of strain on the right ventricle on the ECG. A pulmonary embolus rarely shows changes on an ordinary chest x-ray film and a pulmonary angiogram is required to demonstrate it.

Treatment consists of bed rest and heparin administration. Heparin helps to prevent further spread of clotting in the deep veins and thus helps to minimise the occurrence of emboli.

Occasionally a patient will survive a large embolus long enough to allow it to be removed by surgery. This is a very major operation and is only undertaken when the embolus is thought to be life-threatening.

Good physiotherapy and early ambulation help to reduce the incidence of pulmonary embolism.

Further management of respiratory complications

Any respiratory complication, if severe, may be life threatening and in these circumstances the patient may require to be transferred to the intensive therapy unit (ITU). In the ITU, prolonged respiratory support can be provided including artificial ventilation of the lungs if need be, as well as intensive physiotherapy, tracheal suction, bronchoscopy, etc.

Index